To Claire !
Stay H
♡ Alex   xxx

C000215382

TRANSFORM
FOR LIFE

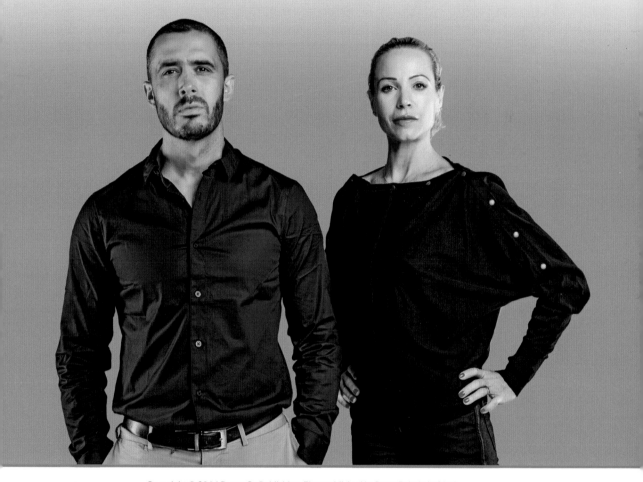

Book designed by R & W Media Limited.
Edited by Nichola Tyrrell, Jo Lightfoot and L. Staggs.
Photography by Lovelight Photography.
Index by Judith Reading.

ISBN: 978-1-9999551-0-6

www.teambodyproject.com

For Zoe.

FOREWORD BY THE AUTHOR

From boxing rings in the dusty backstreets of London to boardrooms in skyscrapers that dominate the city's skies, most of my life has been spent in pursuit of helping people change their bodies.

Therefore, this next statement may surprise you.

I do not think you need to change your body.

For many years this philosophy prevented me from writing this book.

The invigoration of acceptance in mind rather than a pursuit of perfection of body is the more effective route towards lifelong health, and somewhat ironically, a far more stable route towards aesthetic change.

I feared that writing a book which outlined the scientific, anecdotal and observational lessons I have learned around transformative physical change would encourage a focus on an impossible physical perfection – yet I have learned that armed with the facts, people can make the best decisions for themselves.

Transform for Life contains all the information you need about physical change; how you choose to use this information is down to you.

The goal of this book is to help you get the most from your body, free from fluff, conjecture and bias.

Transform for Life is how to do 'weight loss/fat loss' right, with no margin for error and an absolute guarantee of results.

If you want to change your body, you are in the right place.

This book was written for every person around the world who trusts me to help them get healthy and achieve their dreams. You inspire me every day.

This book was written with the support of my beautiful wife Alexandra, who lovingly suffers me. A fact that continues to surprise me.

It was written as children ran around my feet, asking Daddy when he could come and play.

"When I've finished the book" has been said much more often than it should.

It was written while a tiny soul whispered truths that can only be whispered by those who live in your heart, where your eyes can't see them, but your spirit feels them. The truth is a profound water that can put out the flames of judgement.

Every word in this book is the truth, as I have found it.

CONTENT GUIDE

THE SCIENCE OF PHYSICAL TRANSFORMATION

THE ART OF CHANGE

TEAM B O D Y PROJECT

THE BLUEPRINT

INTRODUCTION TO TRANSFORM FOR LIFE

Why a lifetime transformation program?

If you're looking for a quick-fix diet plan that promises you rapid results, this book is not for you.

If you want a super simple 'cookie cutter' plan that doesn't require any thought, *Transform for Life* is probably not for you either.

If your goal is definitive physical changes and long-term compliance, we deal in proven methodology.

To ensure you achieve long-term, sustainable, permanent results, we need to do a little hard work at the beginning by creating your *Health Blueprint* that will set you up for life.

Understanding nutrition, exercise and 'self coaching' is not hard and throughout this experience we will coach you to coach yourself towards lifelong transformative health success.

If you want to change your body for life, there is no better path than the path that is tailor made for you.

Science meets art

Any coach who tells you that science has all the answers, hasn't coached very many people.

Science has the binary answers, but it needs the *Art of coaching* to function effectively in the incalculably complex and sometimes irrational context of the human mind.

A mind armed with 'philosophies' aligned with scientifically proven exercise and nutrition protocols is the environment in which compliance actually happens.

Understanding the habits and philosophies behind compliance and long-term success would be infinitely more important to long-term sustainability than whether you are eating 35% or 40% carbohydrates.

If you've ever struggled with compliance, our *Emotional Eating Handbook* and *The Art of Change* section will be invaluable in your journey.

One final point

The work required to be successful with *Transform for Life* is **front-loaded**.

The next couple of weeks will require you to use your brain, your time, your energy and your discipline. This will set you up to live the rest of your life in the body you want.

You will create your personal *Blueprint*. This *Blueprint* will become more valuable than any diet book or health plan in the world.

Over time, the principles and lessons you learn and implement will become second nature as you develop a healthy relationship with your body and the foods you choose to eat.

WHAT IS THE TRANSFORM FOR LIFE ONLINE PROGRAM?

The information in this book can be applied alongside all exercise and nutrition programs.

However, for a complete *end to end* experience *Transform for Life* is best accompanied by our online exercise and coaching support system at **www.teambodyproject.com** - where you can follow our workout plans, receive our coaching and speak with others taking part from around the world.

The *Transform for Life* program is a fun, interactive and fully supported exercise and nutrition experience. You will discover the best ways to eat and develop a great relationship with health, nutrition and movement.

What does the *Transform for Life* program include?

- Hundreds of full production video workouts that you can follow from the comfort of your home
- Complete nutrition guidance to ensure you get the results you want
- Complete guidance on how to use our workouts to get the best results
- Step by step walkthrough of how to change your body from the inside out
- Real-time support from Team Body Project Founders Daniel and Alexandra Bartlett
- Being part of a team of like-minded people to offer support and accountability
- Emotional eating and mindset fundamentals

Transform for Life is an interactive, immersive health experience with the most complete and fun exercise programme ever created.

What do I need to complete Transform for Life?

To get the best results from *Transform for Life* you will need:

- A minimum of one set of dumb-bells
- An exercise mat
- Access to a laptop, phone, tablet or television to watch your workouts
- Suitable training shoes and exercise clothing for workouts
- A willingness to put hard work in now to reap the benefits for life
- To let go of past habits and build new ones

What happens when I complete the Transform for Life program?

The *Transform for Life* programme does not end when you achieve your results. You will enter an ever-evolving and engaging maintenance phase where exercise and nutrition find a natural balance among other enjoyable aspects of your life.

Those who complete the *Transform for Life* programme have the option to upgrade to Lifetime *Membership* where exercise plans, nutrition guidance, support and fun activities will continue to challenge, engage and excite you.

HOW TO USE TRANSFORM FOR LIFE

There are a few ways you can use *Transform for Life.*

If you are brand new to exercise and healthy eating...

Quick start

Follow our *Quickstart Guide* in *Additional Resources* and get going. (page 259-266)

When first introducing healthy habits you needn't worry about the details and, provided you follow our exercise plans and make small changes, you will see great results.

Refer to this manual

Once you get started, you can refer to this manual to improve your exercise and healthy eating using the chapter guide as a reference.

Hitting a plateau

Most people will hit a point in their health when they want to accelerate results or overcome a plateau. At this point you can follow the *Transform for Life* manual from *The Blueprint* section onwards.

If you have a history of dieting or weight fluctuations...

Read *The Science of Physical Transformation* and *The Art of Change* sections

If you have a history of losing weight and gaining it back, we suggest you read through these sections to understand the psychological and physiological mechanisms of long-term weight management and overall health.

Create Your *Blueprint*

The Blueprint section will help you find a baseline from which you can become successful for life.

Follow *The Plan*

This will help you implement and self coach your own health plan following our crystal-clear guidelines, exercise plans and coaching methods.

Refer back to this book frequently as you move through your health journey

The *Transform for Life* manual is here for you whenever you want to fine tune your plan.

If you want to Transform for Life from the start...

1. Educate yourself

Read *The Science* and *The Art of Change* sections. These sections will provide an understanding of the coaching method and proven theories behind transformative change.

Or skip 1. and go straight to 2:

2. Create your personal blueprint

Follow the path laid out for you from *The Blueprint* onwards and use the guidelines to achieve results.

3. Refer

Use *Transform for Life* to refer back and make changes and improvements to your journey.

THE TRUTH SHALL SET YOU FREE

Facts may be black and white, but the human spirit comes in many shades of grey.

The facts of weight loss and body transformation may be absolute, but your approach to them needn't be.

The purpose of *Transform for Life* is not to create anxiety and obsession around food and exercise, but rather to provide absolute clarity around physiological changes that you can trust.

You will be able to use the information in this book in different ways.

1. Follow every word and **expect** results exactly the way you want them.

2. Follow most of the guidance and **expect** good results.

3. Incorporate a few ideas and **hope** for results – but accept that if they aren't the ones you wanted, that's absolutely fine.

4. Acknowledge the information, decide it doesn't fit your lifestyle, throw away the scales and the measuring tape, rip up this book up and throw it on the fire.

If you want to **guarantee** results, you will need to pick number one or two, but that does not mean it should be your preference or that it is the right answer, or the wrong one.

All options are equals. Even number 4, unless you are reading this on a kindle.

Provided we can make the truth our story, we can use it in any way we choose.

The truth guides us from damaging relationships with false beliefs that keep us circulating in the never-ending cycle of dieting.

While facts can seem harsh on face value, they are liberating when you peer deeper. The diet industry thrives on feeding half truths that convince people there must be a magic way, when there is not.

"Whatever I try, I can't seem to lose weight" can be replaced with a positive decision and philosophy.

"The requirements of weight loss do not suit my lifestyle or preferences, therefore I am going to focus on being healthy and loving my body the way it is."

This is a philosophy I wish more people had. Be healthy and forget the scales and the measuring tape.

Once you are presented with the truth you can make choices that are important to your life, circumstances and expectations.

Drinking a branded protein shake and eating a bucket of superfoods for breakfast, lunch and dinner won't help you if you don't get the fundamentals right.

You might never come within sniffing distance of a supplement or have an avocado pass your lips, provided you implement the fundamentals of change.

With *Transform for Life* I do not seek to persuade you of what is right and what is wrong, just what is true; proven in the lab, in the trenches of professional sport and the battlefields of transformative change.

Once you are in possession of the facts you can make your decision accordingly.

Provided you are armed with the requisite facts, I support them all.

THE SCIENCE
OF PHYSICAL TRANSFORMATION

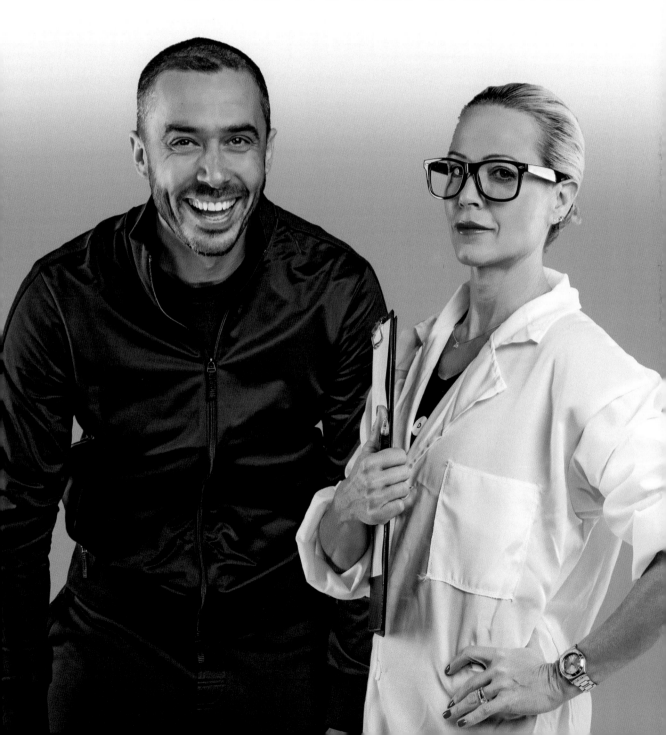

INTRODUCTION TO SCIENCE

Weight loss is incredibly simple, so why the need for an explanation of the science of physical change?

While weight loss is a binary process, healthy, sustainable fat loss and muscle retention is less so, but still easy to implement if you understand the laws that surround it.

These are the laws anybody can apply to ensure results that are:

- Repeatable
- Predictable
- Sustainable

As a sports conditioning coach, I had a very simple task:

- To ensure the athlete made an exact weight by a specific date
- To ensure the athlete retained muscle and lost fat

This precise role removed the margin for error and forced me to let go of preconceived ideas and attach to the evidence-based methods that I have successfully used with hundreds of personal clients and thousands of people around the world.

Every person reading this book can apply these methods to their own body if they are willing to spend time to:

- Understand *The Science* behind this coaching method
- Practise *The Art* of compliance
- Develop a personal *Health Blueprint*

Transform for Life will provide you with every piece of information I have learned from coaching thousands of people, distilled into one short book. The more you understand how your body works, the more exciting you will find the journey you travel with it.

FUNDAMENTALS OF FAT LOSS

This chapter is more than a little 'sciencey' because it has to be.

Read the chapter as many times as you need to bring clarity to the fundamental processes at play when changing your body.

'Eat less, move more' provides more than a degree of truth but, as is often the case, this small amount of knowledge has been a very dangerous thing in the hands of marketers, dieters and professionals alike.

This chapter, and the entire *Transform for Life* method, will help you understand how to lose fat, build muscle and sustain a healthy metabolism.

Fundamental law of weight loss

Weight loss is incredibly simple. The amount of energy we consume is either less than or more than the amount we use. [1,2]

- If we consume fewer calories than we use, we lose total weight. [3]
- If we consume more calories than we use, we gain total weight.
  This is the fundamental law of 'weight loss'. The overall mass of an object is ruled by the total energy it consumes versus the total energy it burns.

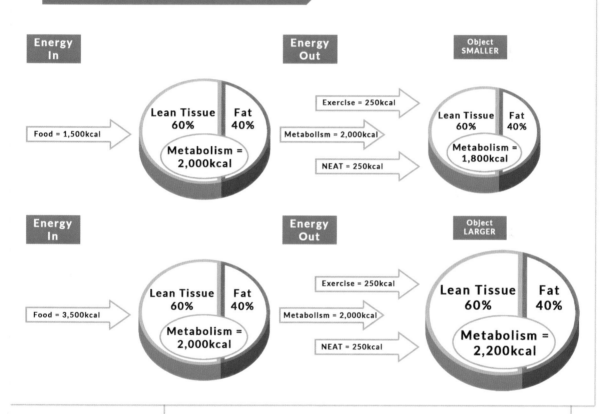

If there is less energy consumed the object will get smaller.
If there is more energy the object will get larger.

Note 1: *Without any consideration of exercise, macronutrients or flux, the object changes size but the composition remains the same.*

Note 2: *The metabolism is slower the smaller the object is, as a smaller object requires less energy to exist.*

Calorie balance is the driving force behind weight loss.

Wrap this information up tight. Store it deep in your mind and remove all potential for doubt. It is not worth reading any more of this book until you have established this certainty.

Superfoods have lots of super qualities, but eat too much of them, you'll have an expanding waistline.

- Avocados may be packed with goodness, but they do not cause you to lose weight.
- Sugar has many negative effects on health, but it does not cause you to gain weight.
- Too few calories cause you to lose weight.
- Too many calories cause you to gain weight.

We cannot avoid this fact, regardless of the complexities that surround weight management discussed throughout this book.

Weight loss happens when we eat less than we burn.

Once we can establish this truth, we free ourselves to focus on more important matters, like fat loss, food quality, body composition and even the seemingly contradictory fact that not all calories are created equal.

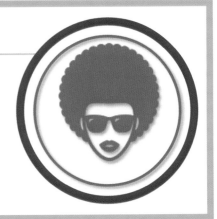

Lily's Laws 1

Lily likes proven facts that help people achieve results.

Whenever Lily hears a universal law of change, she adds it to her list. If she hears nonsense she gets pretty upset, but fortunately that won't happen often here.

Anyway, Lily just found her **FIRST** universal law.

- **Calorie balance drives weight management.**

The basics of body composition

Just eating fewer calories is a binary solution to a complex problem with a number of consequences:

1. We may have lost as much muscle as we did fat. [4]
2. Chronic exposure to calorie deficits may cause negative changes to the metabolism. [5]
3. Chronic exposure to calorie deficits may cause you to feel tired, restricted and lacking in energy. [6]
4. All calories are not created equal (covered later in *Is a calorie a calorie?* Pages 44-51).

Any fat loss plan must be driven by a calorie deficit. However, subtle changes will make the difference between a positive overall experience versus a restrictive and difficult experience resulting in a body that remains too high in relative fat levels.

There are two fundamental caloric states we can be in:

Hypocaloric is a calorie deficit (less than baseline) and hypercaloric is a calorie surplus (more than baseline).

It is almost impossible to have an exact match of '**input versus output**', therefore you are always either:

A.   **Catabolic** – this is a state in which your body breaks down tissue. This is the state in a calorie **deficit (hypocaloric)**.[7]

Or

B.   **Anabolic** – a state in which your body builds and repairs. This is the state in a calorie **surplus (hypercaloric)**. [8]

Catabolic is a state of demolition. The body is destroying and breaking things down.

King Klong and Rob the Builder

When King Klong runs out of food he gets angry!

A **Catabolic** body sets Klong free.

Klong hates stored fat because he can't eat it, so he smashes it up and turns into food he can eat.

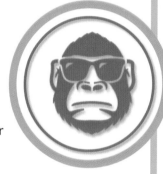

When you eat fewer calories than you are burning you set King Klong free, but remember, Klong gets bored after a while and starts looking for other stuff to smash. Like muscle. He hates muscle because he can't eat that either!

Maybe Klong isn't all that bad. Maybe he doesn't hate things. Maybe Klong just wants to smash things. Everything.

That's why we've got to put Klong back in his cage every now and then.

Anabolic is a building state run by chief builder Rob when you have enough food.

Sometimes Rob the Builder is understandably scared of King Klong, so Rob won't come out of hiding until Klong is safely back in his cage.

Rob just loves building and repairing muscle, but if he's never got any materials to build with, he has no choice but let things go to ruin.

Though, if he's got too many materials, he stores them in fat deposits.

> If Rob has just enough of the right stuff and enough time to do it, he can adapt and repair wonderful muscular buildings!
>
> If you treat Klong and Rob fairly, letting Klong out to smash some fat,
> and letting Rob out to repair some muscle, you can build whatever you like, however you like.
>
> If you overuse either of them, the results can be disastrous.

Together, these two processes make up your metabolism. [9]

Dieting culture features chronic calorie deficits, as calorie deficits result in total weight loss.

Calorie counting, portion control, removal of processed foods, clean eating and every variant of diet that evokes weight loss has identified a route to generating a deficit (hypocaloric state) and the catabolic, fat-burning environment it creates.

What most weight loss plans fail to explain is the following:

A.   It is very unlikely you will build muscle in a calorie deficit. [10]

B.   Chronic or long-term exposure to a calorie deficit will cause you to metabolise muscle. [11, 12, 13]

C.   Long-term exposure to chronic calorie deficits can result in loss of energy, reduced brain function and a drop in baseline metabolic rate. [14, 15]

D.   Rebound eating – the level and/or duration of restriction will drive the dieter towards excessive consumptions to compensate. [16, 17, 18]

This is important information to be aware of before placing yourself in a permanent caloric deficit.

The first goal of any fat loss method should be retention of muscle, as this lean tissue supports a stronger metabolism and improves insulin sensitivity.

Let's assess the different expectations you can have:

1. Calorie surplus, anabolic dominant

a) If you wish to build muscle you should be in a calorie surplus alongside a relevant exercise plan. [19, 20]

b) You will gain fat in a calorie surplus if you are not exercising and/or eating too high a ratio of low-quality foods.

Rob will only build and repair if he has sufficient calories to do so.

2. Calorie deficit, catabolic dominant

a) If you wish to lose fat you should be in a calorie deficit and exercising.

b) You may lose muscle in a calorie deficit if you are not exercising, eating a high ratio of low-quality foods or in a permanent deficit.

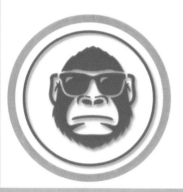

Klong only gets set free from his cage when he runs out of food.

- Your body does not want to build muscle or store fat in a hypocaloric, catabolic state as it does not have an excess energy balance to use.

- Your body does not want to break down muscle or fat in a hypercaloric, anabolic state as it already has enough energy.

The Flux

Flux is a period of higher calories, either individual days or entire weeks, to support anabolic repair and adaptation. [21]

If weight loss is your goal, you can aim to sustain an absolute calorie deficit but introduce a calorie flux to:

- Support muscle repair and retention.
- Avoid down regulation of metabolism.
- Keep energy levels and mental resilience high.
- Avoid cravings, emotional eating and loss of drive.
- Maximise fat loss.

Flux makes the difference between long-term success with healthy body composition rather than the short-term flat weight loss as promised by *ELMM (Eat Less, Move More)*.

In order to lose fat and build/retain muscle you will need to spend the majority of your time in calorie deficit, which will enable fat loss, but to retain and build muscle you will need to spend a shorter, but significant amount time in a calorie surplus.

This significant detail will transform your long-term weight management outlook.

Lily's Laws 2

Good news! Lily just found a **NEW** universal law of change.

- Calorie balance
- **Flux is needed to support anabolic repair and adaptation**
- **Anabolic and catabolic flux**

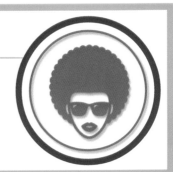

Case study – Elena, 28

Elena had been exercising for 30 minutes a day and eating 1,200 kcal for 12 weeks. At first she had been losing weight, but it slowed down and she suspected she was losing muscle. She was feeling increasingly weaker as the days and weeks went on. Her compliance was slipping and she was no longer enjoying exercise.

Elena was eating less and moving more, but her flat calorie reduction was causing both fat and healthy tissue losses. She had expected to be building muscle, but her body was chronically exposed to a breakdown state.

Flat calorie reductions also impact long-term adherence, as an underfed body will not be an energetic, motivated one.

This physiological change has an influence on psychology and compliance.

By introducing two higher calorie, higher training days per week we were able to help Elena continue to lose weight while retaining and potentially building muscle, and help ensure weight loss was almost exclusively fat.

Previous diet:

- 1,200 calories 7 days per week (100% catabolic), chronic exposure to anabolic state.
- 6 days per week exercise.
- Total caloric intake – 8,400.
- Outcome – slowed metabolism and metabolic processes, less fat loss and more muscle loss, fatigue, loss of strength, cravings, struggles for willpower.

New diet:

- 1,200 calories 5 days per week, 1,500 calories 2 days per week (70% catabolic, 30% anabolic) small calorie flux.
- 4 days per week 30 minutes exercise, 2 days per week 30 minutes exercise + 15 minutes additional resistance.
- Total caloric intake – 9,000.
- Outcome – retained muscle, fat loss, improved strength, metabolic processes retained, high energy, less cravings, higher motivation.

This crucial change transformed Elena's results and the way she felt physically and psychologically throughout her health plan.

The 'excess fat' caveat

When you mobilise fat, you create energy for use. This new energy is released when we free the energy available within stored fat cells. [22]

If we can free energy when we mobilise fat, is it ever truly possible to be in a chronic hypocaloric state if there is 100 lbs of fat in stored, converted energy available to mobilise.

The answer is, it depends.

If your pancreas is functioning well enough to release sufficient amounts of the hormones that mobilise or free fat cells, it is possible your body is in a cycle of creating usable calories from within its stores, and thus generating an anabolic, or building state, from within.

Note: This would require Rob the Builder to not be scared of Klong. Think of Klong throwing fat down for Rob to use. This could happen, but equally it may not, sometimes Rob is just a coward.

Note: We look at this 'metabolic flexibility' in more detail in the next chapter – Carbohydrates and metabolic flexibility. (pages 23-28)

As a rule, the more fat you have to lose, the longer you can stay in a deficit without worrying about losing muscle and potentially gaining fat, but nonetheless, some form of flux remains important to your long-term results.

Protecting metabolism

The difference between a strong, fully functional metabolism and a 'weak' metabolism is estimated to be between 100 and 300 calories.[23]

A slowed metabolism through loss of muscle and protective adaptations is not drastic, but that does not mean it is not significant. Our metabolism naturally slows as we lose weight, so protecting our metabolism where we can is crucial. [24]

A smaller object has lower caloric requirements than a larger one and needs less energy; if you weigh less, you need less. Many people wonder why they stop losing weight on the same level of calories they were consuming when they started a new diet, but this is actually to be expected. [25]

Flat calorie reduction

	A: 200 lb (90 kg) man	B: 150 lb (68 kg) man
Workouts	6 x	6 x
Calories burned per workout	400 kcal	350 kcal
Total calories burned	2,400 kcal	2,100 kcal
Weekly Baseline Metabolic Rate	2,450 kcal x 7	1,950 kcal x 7
Weekly BMR + burn total	19,550 kcal	15, 750 kcal
Calories consumed	15,000 (2,142 per day)	15,000 (2,142 per day)
Weight loss	1-2 lb (0.45-0.9 kg)	0 lb

There is nothing wrong with the metabolism of the 150 lb (68 kg) man (person B), he just doesn't need as much energy because he doesn't have as much total mass. [26]

We can't avoid all slowing in the metabolism as we lose weight, but it is imperative we protect against making it slower than it has to be:

1. Ensuring we retain muscle through regular exercise and sufficient protein consumption.
2. Avoiding unnecessary adaptive changes to the metabolic rate.
3. Building additional muscle during anabolic states.

Muscle is three times more metabolically active at rest than fat. If we can retain muscle, build small amounts of muscle and ensure we are losing as close to 100% fat as possible, we not only support a healthier-looking body, but a more metabolically active one.

We can also avoid slowing of metabolic rate through the use of flux. [27, 28]

If we take the example of person B in this second table we can see the difference a good approach can make.

The differences are not dramatic and would be difficult to note over a week or two. There is no drastic starvation mode, but rather a subtle flux that compounds to ensure long-term maintenance, higher energy, more emotional balance and continued progress are more achievable outcomes.

Our objective when we are losing weight and keeping it off is to mimic the outcome of person B.

	A: 150 lb man, high body fat	B: 150 lb man, low body fat
Daily caloric intake	1,830 kcal	1,830 kcal
Average metabolic rate	1,950 kcal	1,950 kcal
Additional muscle mass	-5 lb -20 kcal	+10 lb +40 kcal
Metabolic strength	Poor -50 kcal	Good +50 kcal
Current metabolic rate	1,880 kcal per day	2,040 kcal per day
Weekly difference	-1,120 kcal	+1,120 kcal
6 months weight difference*	0 lb	8 lb (3.6 kg)
12 month weight difference*	0 lb	16 lb (7.2kg)

We use the slightly dated example of 3,500 kcal = 1 lb of body weight. This is not expected to be entirely accurate but is used as a guideline to provide an example of the difference small changes to metabolic rate and muscle retention makes to long-term weight loss.

There are four key variables to consider within your own plan that are going to impact you:

1. How extreme your calorie deficits and surpluses are.
2. The length of time you spend in each of these states, or more importantly the ratio between one and the other.
3. How much and the type of exercise you do.
4. The macronutrient (carbohydrates, fat and protein) balance you choose.

How you can approach each of these for your own circumstances is covered in the *Transform for Life* journey.

Fundamentals of fat loss recap

Key points:

- A calorie deficit is imperative to overall weight loss.
- Permanent deficits result in potential muscle loss and slowed metabolism.
- A catabolic environment supports fat loss.
- An anabolic environment supports muscle repair and adaptation.
- Flux will help you retain muscle and metabolic strength.
- Flux ratios will be dependent on current body fat and weight.

Things to do:

- Calculate required calories.
- Build in flux days and weeks.
- Monitor weight loss against fat loss, either using measurements or with calipers.

Transform for Life – The Blueprint will help you set your calories and flux correctly.

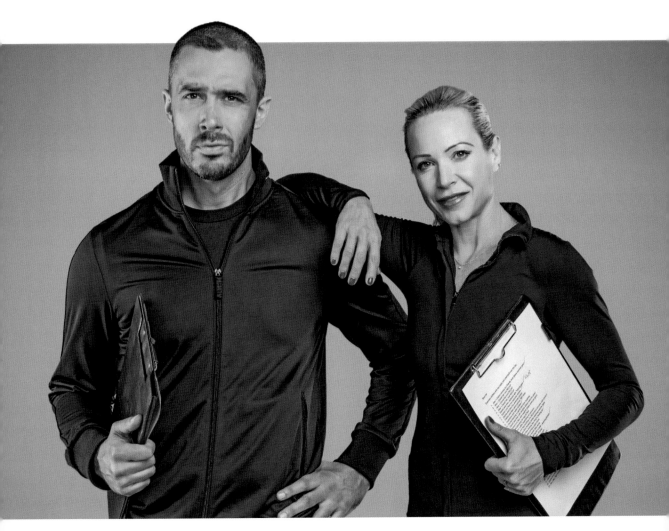

CARBOHYDRATES AND METABOLIC FLEXIBILITY

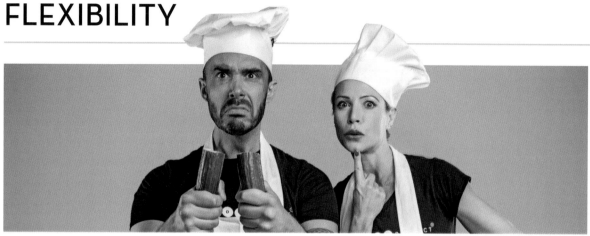

Now we understand the basics of calorie balance and flux, we can start to look at the influence various macronutrients have on our health and physiques.

The truth about carbs

We are surrounded by conflicting information about carbohydrates and it can be difficult to understand the place they have in our overall health plans.

Let's bust a few myths before we break down the science.

1.   Insulin does not make you gain weight. It has a large part to play in body composition and overall health, but limited influence on total weight loss and gain.[1, 2]
2.   Carbohydrates are not good or bad. They are just macronutrients.
3.   Fat doesn't make you fat, nor do carbs. Calories do.

All healthy diets include a balance of protein, fat and carbohydrates. However, a healthy balance for you may be very different from a healthy balance for me.

Lily's Laws 3

Good news! Lily just found a **NEW** universal law of change.

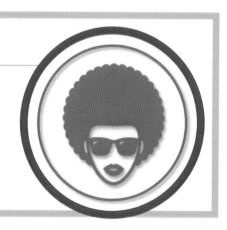

- Calorie balance
- Anabolic and catabolic flux
- **Sufficient carbohydrates are needed in a healthy diet***

*Ketogenic diets (see *Popular diets*) are an exception to this rule.

Think of the body as a post depot

As mail (energy) comes in, different workers (hormones like glucagon and insulin) have different roles to ensure the mail gets to the right place (repair muscle, provide energy). The better trained your workforce (endocrine system) the more different types of mail your depot (body) can cope with.

With a poorly trained workforce, you can only accept certain types of mail (carbohydrates OR fat OR protein).

With an efficiently trained workforce, your body can cope with many different types of mail and confidently ensure they all arrive in the right place.

Our goal is to ensure your body can cope with all types of macronutrients, but it may need some training to get it there.

The transport hormones

Glucagon is a hormone that works alongside insulin. Both are released from the pancreas.

Insulin helps nutrients get INTO the cells and glucagon releases the stored nutrients OUT OF the cells, to be used as energy.

- It is glucagon that releases free fatty acids from your fat stores. [3]
- It is insulin that transports energy to the cells to be used.

A higher release of insulin is important if you wish to build muscle and a higher release of glucagon is important if you wish to lose fat.

Klong and Rob

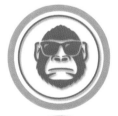

Think of glucagon as the key that sets Klong free from his cage.

Think of insulin as the train that delivers building materials to Rob.

Since both building muscle and burning fat are important to long-term health success, we cannot neglect the importance of either.

Insulin and glucagon are never present at the same time. The pancreas either releases insulin in response to sugar, or releases glucagon in response to protein and fat or a fasted state.[4]

Note: *A fasted state is when the body has no readily available macronutrients of any type.*

The presence of insulin or glucagon is what determines whether food is used as building materials or stored as fat.[5,6]

In an ideal world, your body would move effortlessly between these two pathways, insulin transporting amino acids into muscle cells to help repair, before switching to glucagon when carbohydrates are not available, freeing fat from cells to be converted into energy.

For *metabolically flexible* people, a balanced level of carbohydrates, fat and protein is all that is required to ensure the body is spending time building muscle and burning fat. Since both building muscle and burning fat are important to long-term health success, we cannot neglect the importance of either.

Insulin and glucagon are never present at the same time. The pancreas either releases insulin in response to sugar, or releases glucagon in response to protein and fat or a fasted state.[4]

The presence of insulin or glucagon is what determines whether food is used as building materials or stored as fat.[5,6]

In an ideal world, your body would move effortlessly between these two pathways, insulin transporting amino acids into muscle cells to help repair, before switching to glucagon when carbohydrates are not available, freeing fat from cells to be converted into energy.

For *metabolically flexible* people, a balanced level of carbohydrates, fat and protein is all that is required to ensure the body is spending time building muscle and burning fat.

However, the majority of people are more efficient at releasing insulin in response to carbohydrate consumption than releasing glucagon in response to lowered levels of blood sugar, and converting stored fat to energy. We call this being carb adapted.

As long as there is the possibility of insulin-based energy release, the body will not make much effort to switch to the glucagon fat-releasing pathway.

Rather than switch to glucagon energy release, your body will send urgent hunger signals via your brain to get more carbohydrate for energy release. People talk of the period, two weeks after reducing starchy carbohydrates, when these cravings subside. This is the point at which the body has adapted to the glucagon pathway.

A higher carbohydrate diet can block fat loss in an individual with poor glucagon response. As long as insulin is being released, the body has no reason to switch to glucagon and commence the process of freeing energy from fat cells for energy.

Klong and Rob

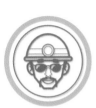

Carb adapted = The body is scared of releasing Klong from his cage and prefers to keep Rob busy.

Fat adapted = Klong is permanently on the rampage and Rob never gets a chance to build anything.

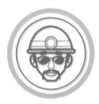

Metabolically flexible = Klong and Rob respect each other and work together effortlessly.

Case study – Aaron, 48

Aaron was confused when I first met him. A book he had read told him that he should eat a balance of carbohydrates. However, a personal trainer friend had told him that carbs were bad.

He had been caught between polarizing viewpoints and felt overwhelmed by the information.

"I was determined to make a change, but was frightened I would make the wrong choice. Should I cut out carbs or would that be bad for me? It's hard to follow through on a plan when you don't know what is right."

I asked Aaron about his food habits over the last few years. His high sugar and carb consumption alongside his pre-diabetic condition told me it was likely his body was not going to cope with high levels of starchy carbohydrates.

For the first six months of his diet, we tracked carefully, keeping him between 25% and 30% carbohydrates, including fibre and starches.

After six months, we started increasing his ratios of carbs and dropping his fat ratios. At this point we found his performance and muscle development started to improve rapidly.

After 12 months, and with 55 lb (25 kg) weight loss, Aaron was on a balanced diet of 40% carbohydrates, 30% fat and 30% protein while continuing to perform well and lose fat. He had developed metabolic flexibility and could enjoy a balanced diet.

Carbs were not and are not bad for Aaron, but their continued presence was preventing his body from making the necessary adaptations.

Factors that increase glucagon production include:

- Diets lower in sugar and starchy carbs
- Exercise
- Eating enough protein
- Fasting/reducing calories

Factors that decrease glucagon production include:

- Frequent meals
- High blood sugar
- Refined carbohydrates
- Sedentary behaviour

The pancreas of a metabolically flexible individual will be able to produce glucagon in the presence of carbohydrate consumption because their pancreas does not see one pathway as preferable to the other and will respond based on current nutrient availability.

Neither insulin nor glucagon are inherently bad, it is overexposure to one or the other that can cause some problems.

Knowing that muscle growth and retention is responsible for metabolic strength, performance and aesthetic appearance, even when fat loss is the goal, insulin remains an important component of any permanent health plan.

What we can learn

Consider your diet history.

- Have starchy carbohydrates been a mainstay of your diet?
- Do you binge on carbohydrates?
- Are your cravings carbohydrate-based?

You may be carb adapted and need to reduce carbs in the short-term to rebalance the way your body works and ensure fat loss.

A long-term goal is to have a balanced intake of carbohydrates, fat and protein, but training your body to switch energy systems by temporarily reducing carbohydrate ratios in the short-term is an effective strategy.

Conclusion

Carbohydrates are not bad, but they could be interfering with your fat loss goals right now.

We will help you find your correct carbohydrate ratios in the *Transform for Life – The Blueprint* section.

Carbohydrates and metabolic flexibility recap

Key points:

- Insulin transports energy to cells – both muscle and fat. Without insulin, building muscle is extremely tough.
- Glucagon helps mobilise fat for energy use, making it an important hormone.
- Carb adapted individuals may struggle to produce glucagon and therefore lose fat with higher carb diets.
- Neither carbs nor insulin are inherently bad, but they may be bad for your goals right now.
- Long-term expectations should include balanced carbohydrate levels for most people.

Things to do:

- Consider your diet history and whether lower carbs may be suitable.
- Choose a starting carbohydrate ratio accordingly.
- Monitor outcomes and update.

Transform for Life – The Blueprint will help you get the starting carbohydrate ratio right for you.

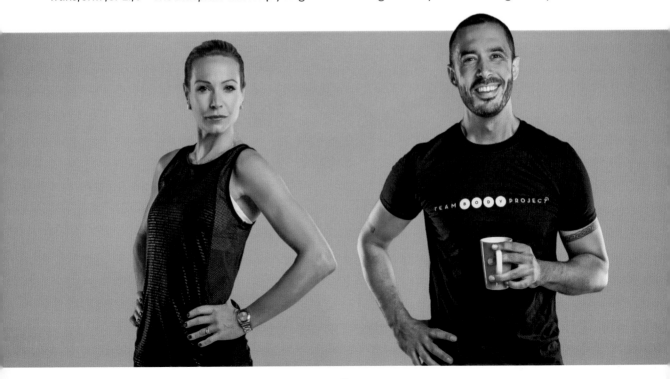

THE ROLE OF PROTEIN

If carbohydrates and fats provide us with energy, proteins provide us with building blocks to repair and build our muscles.

To achieve our health goals, sufficient protein consumption is essential.

The building blocks of life

Proteins are the building blocks of life. Everything we are and everything we will become is moulded with protein-infused bricks.

Protein builds and repairs muscle that supports a strong metabolism. [1,2]

Without adequate dietary protein, the body will resort to utilising protein from the retained pools within our muscles. For this reason, ensuring ample protein is available at all times is crucial when transforming our bodies.

Klong and Rob

When Rob notices the body isn't getting enough dietary protein, he shouts to Klong (from the safety of HQ) to start smashing down muscle cells instead of fat cells.

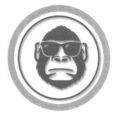

Klong likes smashing things, so he's happy to oblige. Even if he secretly thinks Rob is a goody two shoes.

Your protein baseline

Protein levels should not fluctuate much once we have found our baseline, and these levels will typically hold regardless of whether we are dropping or increasing calories.

While a sufficient level of protein is paramount for muscle retention and growth, an excess of protein provides very little benefit in exchange for numerous potential problems. [3]

Finding the correct levels of protein for you is one of the challenges you will face early on in creating your *Health Blueprint*.

Too little protein and you run the risk of losing muscle, too much and you run the risk of turning the excess into glucose via gluconeogenesis and storing it as fat.

Around 0.7-1.2 g of protein per pound (1.54-2.64g per kg) of body weight is a safe starting point, more with high levels of resistance training and less if your exercise levels are low.*

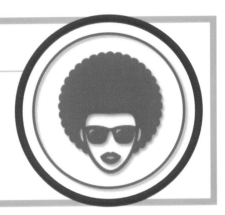

Lily's Laws 4

Good news! Lily just found a **NEW** universal law of change.

- Calorie balance
- Anabolic and catabolic flux
- Sufficient carbohydrates
- **Sufficient protein is needed to ensure muscle repair and adaptation**

*_**Note:** If you considerably increase your levels of resistance training or circuit training, you will also be increasing the demand on the body to repair/build muscle tissue and therefore also increasing the quantity of protein required._

Conversely, if you reduce the amount of resistance and circuit training, it may be worth considering reducing your protein consumption, but again, only by a small amount.

Protein and calorie deficits

An incremental increase in relative protein in a calorie deficit is useful in almost all instances. The increase in relative protein is created through protecting the protein intake as calories drop rather than by increasing the total protein levels.

Example:
You can see that while the ratio of protein changes from 30% to 40% in the lower calorie diet, the absolute amount of protein remains at 0.8 g per pound (1.76 g per kg) of body weight.

Macronutrients based on a 2,000 kcal diet with sufficient protein in 190 lb (86 kg) female:

Macronutrients	Calories	Ounces/Grams	% ratio
Proteins	**600 kcal**	**5 oz / 150 g***	**30%**
Fats	600 kcal	2 oz / 67 g	30%
Carbohydrates	800 kcal	7 oz / 200 g	40%

* 0.8 g of protein per pound (1.76 g per kg) of body weight.

Weight loss (hypocaloric) macronutrients based on 1,600 kcal diet with sufficient protein in 190 lb (86 kg) female:

Macronutrients	Calories	Ounces/Grams	% ratio
Proteins	**600 kcal**	**5 oz / 150 g***	**40%**
Fats	500 kcal	2 oz / 55 g	30%
Carbohydrates	500 kcal	4 oz / 125 g	30%

* 0.8 g of protein per pound (1.76 g per kg) of body weight.

When we move our bodies into a calorie deficit, the first action is to protect our protein intake. In a deficit, we are better to go above our protein ratio than go below our ratio and risk muscle loss.

This is for two reasons:

1. When in a caloric deficit, the body will convert excess or unneeded protein into glucose for energy via a process called gluconeogenesis. [4]

2. Protein has a higher thermic effect than carbohydrates, contributing to calorie deficit goals.

Note: *While a person with higher levels of fat has lower demands for total macronutrients, as they have more retained energy to convert, there remains an equal demand for proteins needed for repair and adaptation.*

Case study – Mark, 39

Mark was becoming frustrated by his loss of strength, relative to his weight loss. He had lost around 20 lb (9 kg) and had a further 80 lb (36 kg) he wanted to lose, yet didn't want to continue to feel weaker as time went on. Despite his weight loss and regular training, he was not happy with the shape his body was taking on.

We found that less than 20% of his total calories were coming from protein sources.

With the five days a week of intense training Mark was doing, this was not nearly sufficient to rebuild his muscles, let alone build new muscle.

I explained to Mark that because he had a high level of stored fat, I had less concern about his energy balance from energy substrates (carbohydrates and fats) than I did from protein.

A lower ratio of dietary protein, paired with high levels of training, had created an environment where his body had been forced to mobilise stored protein. In other words, he was losing muscle instead of fat.

By liberally increasing his dietary protein to 40%, reducing carbs by 15% and fats by 5%, we were able to ensure his body had sufficient protein for repair and therefore any mobilised sources would be those suitable for energy use.

After this protein update, we tracked his fat loss and noted almost 100% of his weight loss was from unwanted fat sources over an eight-week period.

In the case of an individual who wishes to lose fat, the optimum outcome is the conversion of the pool of retained fat into energy, alongside the retention of muscle.

To do this, we must have sufficient dietary protein for repair, otherwise the retained amino acids in our muscles could be converted for use.

When an individual in a calorie deficit has a higher fat percentage, the levels of protein in the diet can be considerably more liberal, as the excess protein will be converted into glucose and burned as fuel.

In the leaner individual, higher levels of protein must be supported by a higher level of fat and carbohydrates. In this instance we recommend smaller calorie deficits to avoid risking muscle loss.

Regardless of these details, anybody who is exercising and in a calorie deficit should have a proportionately higher level of total dietary protein to maximise fat loss and muscle retention. I have rarely seen examples where less than 30% protein (0.7 g per pound or 1.54 g per kg of body weight) is optimal for fat loss in a calorie deficit.

Protein and calorie surpluses

When in a calorie surplus, the demands on protein are less as the total availability of carbohydrates and fats are higher. Carbohydrates act in a protein-sparing manner, allowing the available dietary protein to be used for building new tissue and/or repairing old tissue rather than as an alternative energy source.[5]

In this calorie surplus, 'leftover' calories will typically be the ones that are most difficult to utilise for energy, which are protein. The 'leftover' protein-based calories will be sent to work building new muscle.[6]

This is why carbohydrates, rather than proteins, are increased when moving into a calorie surplus.

In a calorie deficit some of our dietary protein will inevitably be converted into glucose for energy. On the other hand, in a calorie surplus, thanks to higher availability of carbohydrates and fats, the majority of our dietary protein can work exclusively on repairing and building new muscle.

Protein availability

Some researchers believe the **total** amount of protein you consume is less important than a consistent **availability** of protein in the diet.[7]

There is ongoing and inconclusive debate over how much dietary protein we can actually utilise in any given day, and the only thing established with certainty is that this number is not the same for everybody. However, there can be no doubt about the need for a consistent availability of sufficient dietary protein for repair and adaptation.

Klong and Rob

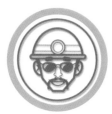

Rob can only do so much building and repairing. He's not magic.

Whenever Klong is safely in his cage and Rob comes out, Rob works as hard as he can, but he can only do so much. If he has surplus protein, he may send the excess off to be converted into energy for other purposes (he may be bright enough to hold some back, but then again he may not be!).

When he comes back to work again, the excess protein from before has been used, so if no new protein has arrived, he sits around doing nothing, or worse, asks Klong to smash some muscles.

All Rob really wants is enough protein to do his job every time he has to do it. You can help out by eating a little protein with every meal.

This is why a plant-based diet can work exceptionally well, even when the total amount of protein is not as high as in meat eating diets.

Most vegans and vegetarians understand the importance of including protein sources in every meal and snack to ensure muscle retention and fat burn.

'Good' versus 'bad' protein availability

Good protein availability

Meal	Protein	Availability
Breakfast	0.7 oz (20 g)	Good
Snack	0.7 oz (20 g)	Good
Lunch	1.1 oz (30 g)	Good
Snack	0.7 oz (20 g)	Good
Dinner	1.1 oz (30 g)	Good
Total	4 oz (120 g)	Moderate

Bad protein availability

Meal	Protein	Availability
Breakfast	0.2 oz (5 g)	Poor
Snack	0 oz	Very poor
Lunch	3 oz (75 g)	Too high
Snack	0.35 oz (10 g)	Good
Dinner	2.1 oz (60 g)	Too high
Total	5 oz (150 g)	High

In the first example we see lower total protein but even availability throughout the day, ensuring that whenever the body needs protein, it is available.

In the second example we see higher total protein, but less even availability throughout the day.

This could force the body to metabolise muscle even though the total amount throughout the day is sufficient. How much does this matter? You will get a different answer depending on who you ask; I prefer to play it safe and ensure sufficient protein throughout the day.

Protein availability versus meal frequency

When it comes to weight loss we have a battle we are continuously fighting.

Ensuring fat loss while protecting against muscle loss

On the one hand, if we continue to feed our body at regular intervals with energy-rich food, we may never force it into the catabolic, glucagon-releasing environment required to free fat cells for energy use. Never feeling hungry means our body may never need to locate alternative energy sources.

On the other hand, if we don't ensure we are providing the body with sufficient protein for repair, we run the risk of muscle loss.

Ensuring the meals and snacks you do have are filled with sufficient protein is your first line of attack, your strongest defence and your greatest ally in improving your body composition.

The role of protein recap

Key points:

- Protein is a building material. We cannot repair and build without it.
- Exercise increases the demands on protein.
- Consuming a protein excess is more of a concern in hypercaloric states than hypocaloric states.
- In order to safeguard current muscle, higher relative protein becomes more critical the further into a hypocaloric state you go.
- Consistent protein availability is potentially as important as total protein consumption.
- The vast majority of protein consumed will be for repair. Even in a surplus, your body is only capable of building very small amounts of muscle. Upping protein considerably once you have established a dietary minimum is at best pointless and at worst detrimental.

Things to do:

- Consume protein with every meal.
- Consume higher relative protein levels when in a hypocaloric deficit.
- When increasing calories, increase carbohydrate or fat levels NOT protein levels unless you have reason to believe your protein levels are too low **or** you are increasing resistance training.
- Aim for between 0.7-1.2 g of protein per pound (1.54-2.64g per kg) of body weight.

Transform for Life – The Blueprint will help you set your starting protein levels.

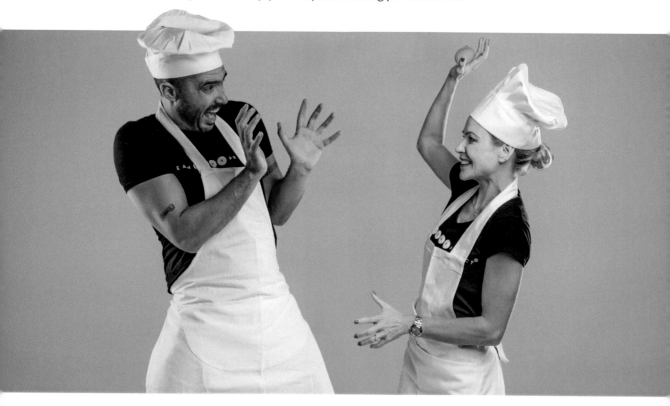

FATS AND RATIOS

Fat is essential.

- It is an alternative and usable form of energy, both as dietary and stored fat.
- It is essential to fight inflammation.
- It is crucial for brain function.
- It is critical for protecting your vital organs.

In the 1970s and 80s, much like carbohydrates are now, fats were demonised, yet we've come to understand how important they are to our existence.

Protein is essential for building and repair, carbohydrates are essential for providing energy, and fat is essential for fighting inflammation, brain function, protecting vital organs and as a potential energy source.

We need all three.

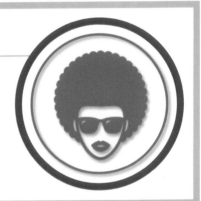

Lily's Laws 5

Good news! Lily just found a **NEW** universal law of change.

- Calorie balance
- Anabolic and catabolic flux
- Sufficient carbohydrates
- Sufficient protein
- **Sufficient fat is needed for brain function, immunity and protection**

The question is not whether we need them, but how much of each we need, and why?

Fat or carbohydrates?

Insulin is often blamed for weight gain because it is responsible for carrying excess energy to be stored in fat cells.

This is the most shocking example of 'shooting the messenger' you are ever likely to hear.

A person gains weight because they eat an excess of calories, the insulin is simply the mail guy.

Without an excess of calories you cannot gain weight. Insulin is not responsible.

It doesn't matter how much insulin you release, if you are in a calorie deficit, your body cannot gain any weight.

However, when it comes to body composition there is more to consider than just the amount of calories we consume. Your macronutrient ratio will play a role in how much fat your body loses.

Knowing that protein is essential for repairing muscles, and levels should remain relatively stable, we are left with a question to answer.

What percentage of our dietary calories should come from fat and how much from carbohydrates?

Higher fat or higher carbs?

Lowering carbohydrates results in a drop in insulin and a rise in glucagon. [1]

Glucagon is needed for freeing stored fat for use and insulin is needed for storing fat. If we look at it from this simple vantage it would seem obvious that dropping carbohydrates would make sense, but we need to look further.

Energy from fat is made available through a longer process of emulsification via digestive processes in the stomach, pancreas and gall bladder.

Once this process is complete, fat is available to be used for specific roles that only fat can complete, while any excess is made available for conversion to energy.

Many tissues, including your muscles, can use fatty acids for energy, but your brain can't convert fatty acids to fuel (unless you enter ketosis, at which point your liver produces ketones – covered in *Popular diets* - pages 67-80). [2]

The brain is a pretty important organ, so if you lower carbohydrates to the extent that your body does not have sufficient usable energy to fuel brain function, your body will simply convert stored or dietary protein into glucose instead. [3]

This process will release insulin and block glucagon production:

A.	Negating the supposed benefits of lower dietary fat by releasing insulin anyway.
B.	Using dietary protein that was meant to repair and regenerate.
C.	Running the 'worst case scenario' risk of metabolising muscle for energy. [4]

This is not to say lowering carbohydrate ratios and raising fat ratios is a bad idea, just that removing carbohydrates and increasing fat will not mean you remove insulin from the equation entirely, and even if you do, it may not be positive.

Note: *We avoid this worst case scenario by ensuring we have macronutrient minimum at all times.*

Whether you have lower carbohydrates or lower fats should be based on numerous factors and is dependent on your current circumstances, goals and even body type. This is all covered in *The Blueprint – Getting started with nutrition.*

Having minimum levels of both fat and carbohydrates is crucial to your long-term function. Beyond this, the fat-to-carbohydrate ratio you consume can be based on the following chart:

Carbs/Fats Ratios

Factor	Ratio change
Fat loss as a goal	Carbs down ↓ fats up ↑
Performance as a goal	Carbs up ↑ fats down ↓
Muscle building as a goal	Carbs up ↑ fats up ↑
Current body fat high	Carbs down ↓ fats up ↑
Current body fat low	Carbs up ↑ fats down ↓

The benefits of lower carb ratios:

- A higher ratio of the fat-burning hormone glucagon is released, meaning more fat should be burned.
- A lower ratio of the fat-storing hormone insulin is released, meaning less fat should be stored.

The benefits of lower fat ratios:

- The brain has sufficient usable energy from carbohydrates to feed the brain and retain dietary protein for repair and adaptation rather than conversion to glucose.
- The body produces enough insulin to be anabolic and build new tissue.
- Performance and energy levels when exercising are better.

Fat and carbohydrate ranges

When you are looking to lose fat as your goal, neither fat nor carb intake should drop below 25% or go above 50%.

Baseline protein in any calorie deficit would rarely be recommended at less than 30% of total calorie intake, leaving you with the remainder to distribute across your energy macronutrients.

Available variable ratio for fat loss goal

- Baseline minimum consumption (fat and carbs): 25% each.
- Minimums total (fat and carbs combined): 50% Protein minimum: 30%+.
- Available variable range: up to 20% (less if protein is higher).

Not enough to make or break your results but enough for you to play with.

Positives and negatives of macronutrient

If you eat just the **minimum of 25% carbohydrates**:

Negatives

- Your performance may suffer.
- You may feel demotivated and tired.

Positives

- You will release more glucagon and may burn a higher percentage of stored fat.
- If you are carb adapted it will help you become metabolically flexible.

If you eat just the **minimum of 25% fats**:

Negatives

- You may release too much insulin, theoretically limiting fat loss.
- You may have more cravings.

Positives
- Your performance should be better.
- You should have more dietary-available protein for use on muscle repair (less need for gluconeogenesis).

What you have hopefully concluded by this point, is:

1.   There is no right answer to which ratio of fats and carbs you should use beyond meeting your minimum requirements on all macronutrients.[5]

2.   There are other factors more important and influential to your overall results than small variables on your macronutrients.

However, just because it is not as significant as other factors, it doesn't mean we should neglect it; the closer we get to reaching our goals, the more important these factors will become.

The following three examples highlight how we can change our macronutrients very slightly, throughout the week, dependent on our specific goals.

Examples of sensible macronutrient ratios based on a 1,500 calorie intake.

1. High protein ratio

This ratio would be suitable on days when you have a higher percentage of resistance training and your priority is muscle repair.

Macronutrients	Calories	Ounces/Grams	% ratio
Proteins	600 kcal	5.3 oz (150 g)	40%
Fats	450 kcal	1.7 oz (50 g)	30%
Carbohydrates	450 kcal	3.9 oz (112.5 g)	30%

2. High fat / low carb ratio

This ratio you may be suitable for days when you are not training and want to limit excess insulin and promote glucagon production.

Macronutrients	Calories	Ounces/Grams	% ratio
Proteins	525 kcal	4.6 oz (130 g)	35%
Fats	600 kcal	2.3 oz (67 g)	40%
Carbohydrates	375 kcal	3.3 oz (94 g)	25%

3. High carb / low fat ratio

This ratio may be better suited to days when you are training hard and need extra carbohydrates for energy.

Macronutrients	Calories	Ounces/Grams	% ratio
Proteins	525 kcal	4.6 oz (130 g)	35%
Fats	375 kcal	1.4 oz (41 g)	25%
Carbohydrates	600 kcal	5.3 (150 g)	40%

Try a ratio:

1. If it works (lose fat, feel good, train well) stick with it.
2. If it doesn't work (don't lose fat, don't feel good, train badly) change it.

None of these ratios would have a dramatically different impact on body composition provided you remain in your calorie deficit, however, as you get closer to your final goal, small differences such as these can become crucial.

All of the above ratios are effective to achieve results, when paired with the key body composition factors and sufficient hydration.

Lily's Laws 6

Good news! Lily just found a **NEW** universal law of change.

- Calorie balance
- Anabolic and catabolic flux
- Sufficient carbohydrates
- Sufficient protein
- Sufficient fat
- **Drink enough water**

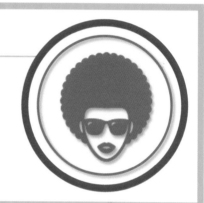

Other points around fats

Essential fatty acids

Omega 6 and omega 3 are essential fatty acids because our body cannot synthesise them, so they have to be ingested.[6]

Provided you are eating a good balance of fats you should not be too concerned, but vegans often need to pay particular caution to omega 3 and sometimes find supplementation can be helpful.

How much fat can you consume at once?

Some people feel sick when they eat high levels of fat, others follow ketogenic diets of 70% or more fat and some people don't even have a gall bladder.

This is where personalisation comes in and why you must not assume any rule is true for you until you have tried it yourself.

Types of fats

There are three types of good dietary fats we need and one we should try to avoid.

Monounsaturated fats and polyunsaturated fats are found in nuts, seeds and oils – these can be around two thirds of our fat source.

Saturated fats can be found in oils and animal products. There is nothing wrong with saturated fats, the problem is they often make up too high a proportion of our diet. Provided they don't make up more than one third of our fats, they are perfectly healthy.

Trans fats found in fried, baked and snack foods are not considered good for our health and should be consumed in small quantities only. They raise the risk of heart disease, raise cholesterol and contribute to insulin resistance. These should be avoided as much as possible. [7]

Does the ketogenic diet work for fat loss?

If your solitary focus is fat loss, a ketogenic diet, where your fat is raised to above 70%, can help you lose fat at a fairly rapid pace.

Fast fat loss is one reason why ketogenic diets have become a popular solution.

A ketogenic diet replaces carbs with dietary fats. People often believe that they are following a ketogenic diet, but fail to get anywhere near the 70% minimum fat levels required to correctly follow this protocol.

This elimination of carbs, along with a relatively low level of protein, largely removes the hormone insulin, replacing it with the glucagon production. Provided you are in a caloric deficit, you can be confident you are burning a proportion of fat because glucagon is the hormone responsible for freeing fats from their cells to use for energy.

After a period of time, the pancreas secretes ketones into the bloodstream, which are able to support fat-fueled brain function and other processes in the absence of blood sugars. [8]

However, ketogenic diets are not without their problems. They are considered to be potentially dangerous for certain populations, especially, but not limited to, diabetics and those with liver or kidney problems.

Our stance is to look for longer, more sustainable habits, but the ketogenic approach can be useful if it suits the individual.

We cover ketogenic diets in a little more detail in *Popular diets*. (pages 67-80)

Fats and ratios recap

Key points:

- Fat is crucial for our immune system, brain function and organ protection.
- Fat ratios should be higher if fat loss is the overall goal.
- Carb ratios should be higher if performance is the overall goal.
- No macronutrient ever needs to be lower than 25% for overall health.
- No macronutrient needs to be higher than 50% for overall health.

Things to do:

- Consider your goals and preferences.
- Try different ratios on high training days to low training days.
- Listen to your body and be flexible with your ratios over time.

Transform for Life – The Blueprint will help you get the starting carbohydrates right for you.

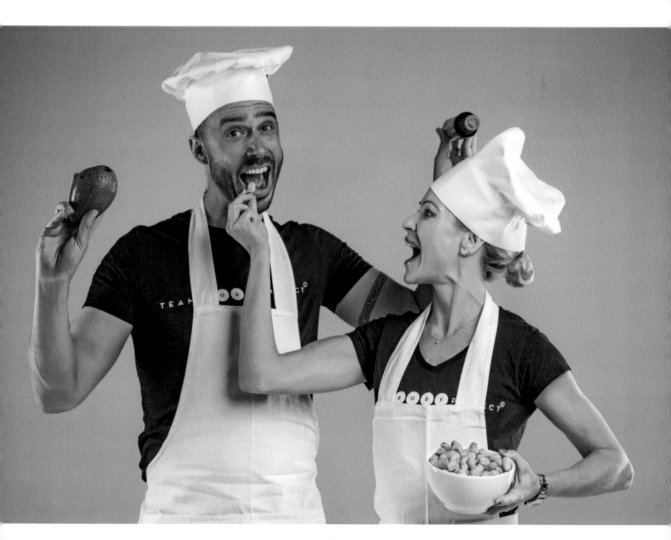

IS A CALORIE A CALORIE?

The scale DOESN'T know how much better you feel and how much energy you have.

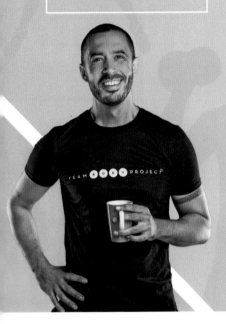

The scale can give you one piece of information and one piece of information only. Your calorie balance.

The scale can tell you whether you have burned more calories than you have consumed or consumed more calories than you have burned.

The scale doesn't know how strong you are, or how great it feels to use your hard-earned muscles.

The scale doesn't know how you can now climb a flight of stairs without being out of breath, or run with your children in the park.

The scale doesn't know about the wonderful way your body is responding to the healthy foods you are eating.

The scale doesn't know how much better you feel and how much energy you have.

The scale doesn't know about the new-found efficiency in your lungs or the extra power that bounds within your every heartbeat.

The scale can tell you whether you have burned more calories than you have consumed or consumed more calories than you have burned.

That is all the scale knows.

No factor is more important than calorie balance for weight loss, but that does not mean all calories are created equally.

Thermodynamics applied to the human body is a different beast from thermodynamics applied in a Petri dish. Different types of calories behave differently within our body, creating vastly different outcomes.

At its simplest level, creating a calorie imbalance explains why we gain weight, but calorie type explains why we might choose to eat more calories in the first place.

Calories and the satiety factor

The hormone ghrelin is responsible for telling you when you are hungry, and the hormone leptin, is responsible for telling you when you are full.

An overall focus on non-processed foods may bring these hormones into balance and make judging fullness and hunger an easier experience, but beyond this, some calories just make us feel fuller than others. [1]

Calorie density looks at the amount of calories per pound and grades the food based on the quantity of calories per pound of food. Calorie density is considered to be strongly, although not absolutely, linked to satiety. [2]

Calorie dense foods:

Food	Calories per pound
Oils	4,000
Nuts and seeds	2,500 – 3,500
Sugars and highly processed carbs	1,500 – 2,000
Breads	1,000 – 1,400
Fish, meats and poultry	400 – 900
Beans and lentils	300 – 750
Potatoes, yams and rice	300 – 600
Fruit	150 – 400
Vegetables	50 – 200

What does this mean?

If you could 'stomach' half a pound of oil it would add up to 2,000 kcal.

The same 2,000 kcal would be up to 40 pounds of food in vegetables.

To eat 2,000 kcal of oils would take you less than a minute, whereas to eat 2,000 kcal of vegetables would take you most of the day.

The increased thermic effect (covered later in this chapter) required through digestion, chewing and continuously lifting the fork when eating vegetables would be significant in this extreme example, but the main difference would actually be on hunger.

The vegetables take up lots of volume in the digestive tract, literally filling the stomach, whereas the oil, despite being heavy on calories, takes up very little space in the digestive tract, leaving our stomach feeling empty. [3]

Even when ignoring the quite significant difference in thermogenesis, the person consuming oil would almost certainly end up eating considerably more calories than the person eating vegetables based on the lack of satiety and fullness they would experience in comparison.

How important is calorie density to your results?

Calorie density and satiety has a place and a part to play in physical change but it is less important than calorie balance and macronutrient ratio.

If you decided weight loss was your only goal and everything else was irrelevant, calorie density would serve you well for a time, but a pure focus on calorie density with no consideration given to macronutrients could end up causing nutritional deficiencies and stalling results.

However, there are lessons to be learned:

- Sugars and processed foods offer little nutritional benefits or calorie density.
- Loading your plates with vegetables is always a good idea.

Lily's Laws 7

Good news! Lily just found a **NEW** universal law of change.

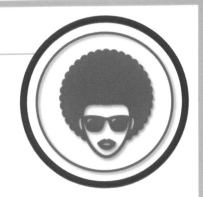

- Calorie balance
- Anabolic and catabolic flux
- Sufficient carbohydrates
- Sufficient protein
- Sufficient fat
- Drink enough water
- **Eat plenty of vegetables**

The thermic effect of food

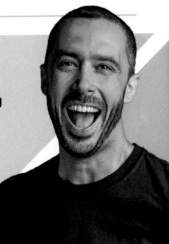

Hot food

The thermic effect of food can be hard to explain. For several minutes I'd been trying to get the concept over to my dad, explaining the delicate interplay between food, heat and metabolism.

Confident I'd got the concept across to him, I asked him to describe it back.

"Son," he said in his thick Cockney brogue, "don't you tell me about the thermic effect of food. I've been eating Vindaloos since before you were born."

Some calories are not equal when it comes to energy balance.

The thermic effect of food measures how the different digestion and metabolising processes of nutrients impact energy expenditure.

Foods travel through different metabolic processes that have varying levels of efficiency. The metabolic processes for protein are less efficient than those for carbs and fats – positive in the context of thermogenics!

If we compare an 1,800 kcal diet with a high protein ratio against an 1,800 kcal diet with a low protein ratio, we can see the difference the higher protein (more thermic) diet has on our overall calorie balance.

Comparison of thermic effect*

	40% high protein	Thermic effect	25% low protein	Thermic effect
Protein	720	180	450	112
Fat	630	19	630	19
Carbs	450	34	720	54
Total calories	1,800	1,800	1,800	1,800
Calories after thermogenesis		1,567		1,615

Based on the following thermic effects: protein 25%, carbs 7.5%, fats 3%

The difference to total calorie intake based on a high protein diet is around 50 kcal.

Is this number worth pointing out? Yes.

Should this impact your decision of how much protein to eat? No.

High protein diets have a metabolic advantage, but this advantage is not sufficient to conflict with our personal preferences and goal-based requirements.

Calorie absorption

The amount of calories we consume is not always the amount of calories we absorb and use. [4, 5]

There are numerous processes involved in the digestion of food; the harder it is to digest food, the less likely we are to extract 100% of the calories from it.

Processed foods are particularly easy for our bodies to digest, therefore we are more likely to absorb and use a higher percentage of calories from them.

Unprocessed, whole foods have a higher fibre and nutrient density and are harder to digest, making it likely that we absorb a lower percentage of calories from them.

Since cooking is a process – foods that are eaten raw are also less likely to be 100% absorbed than foods that are cooked.

Without wanting to paint too vivid a picture, if you don't utilise the calories that go 'in' they still get 'out' again, in the form of excretion. This can, understandably, make the 'in versus out' calculation a little confusing.[6]

It is also the reason some people claim 'clean eating' is more effective for weight loss. 2000 kcal of 'clean' food may result in fewer calories absorbed than 2000 kcal of non 'clean' foods. More on this is available in *Popular diets*.

On top of this, some people absorb more calories than others.

If you and I both ate a 150 kcal egg, it is unlikely both of us would extract 150 kcal of energy from the egg. Perhaps I would absorb 135 kcal and you would absorb 130 kcal.

Despite eating the same amount of food, we can absorb different amounts of calories from that food.

What does this mean? A lot and not very much at all. In fact, it is far more likely to cause you to eat not enough than to eat too much.

When should you worry?

Losing more than 2 lb of weight per week would be a red flag, as would loss of energy, motivation and increased stress levels. If you are maintaining or gaining weight, your absorption levels are not a concern.

If you are losing too much weight, losing energy or feeling uncharacteristically weak, you should eat a higher level of calories than would otherwise be recommended and/or reduce your levels of training.

Provided you are eating a high enough ratio of quality foods, consuming sufficient protein and other macros and regularly exercising, absorption, although impacting, should not be a huge concern for weight or fat loss. You can reduce your levels of absorption by increasing your quantity of whole unprocessed and raw foods – this is a good idea, but wouldn't be recommended in isolation and for the sole purpose of reducing absorption.

Because of factors such as variable absorption, calories in versus calories out cannot be a perfect equation, but it is still the best equation – unless you live in a science laboratory you can never know exactly how many calories you've consumed, absorbed and burned, but over time you can paint a very accurate picture, regardless of important, but secondary factors like absorption rate.

Nutrient quality

The nutrient quality of a food is the amount of vitamins, minerals, fibre and micronutrients within a food.

200 kcal of white bread is not the same as 200 kcal of brown rice, despite having almost identical properties from a macronutrient perspective.

	White bread	Brown rice
Calories	200	200
Carbs	40 g	40 g
Protein	6 g	6 g
Fats	2 g	2 g
Sodium	360 mg	10 mg
Sugar	3 g	1 g
Dietary fibre	1.2 g	4 g

From a calorie and energy perspective, the two products are identical, so when we consider weight loss they are the same, but beyond the obvious increase in sodium, there are two key differences:

1. Dietary fibre is almost 3 g higher in the brown rice.
2. Sugar is 2 g higher in the white bread.

Dietary fibre is important for digestive health alongside numerous other health reasons and most of us don't get enough of it. Dietary fibre slows down the process of digestion, meaning the energy available is distributed more evenly with the brown rice.

On the other hand, sugar digests more rapidly, creating insulin spikes and more readily available glucose. When the body has the deadly combination of insulin and oversupply of available glucose, fat cells become the dumping ground, regardless of whether you are in a surplus or a deficit.

While this example is only a small portion of each product, if this type of decision was made continuously:

- Fat levels would increase
- Insulin sensitivity would decrease
- Hunger would increase
- Satiety would decrease

The vitamins, minerals and micronutrients in the foods we eat are essential in creating health and reducing chances of disease. By limiting processed foods and focusing on a diet that is high in vitamins and minerals we improve every aspect of our health.

Lily's Laws 8

Good news! Lily just found a **NEW** universal law of change.

- Calorie balance
- Anabolic and catabolic flux
- Sufficient carbohydrates
- Sufficient protein
- Sufficient fat
- Drink enough water
- Eat plenty of vegetables
- **Limit processed food intake**

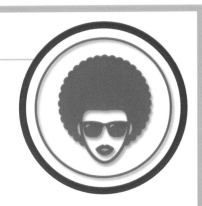

Glycemic index and glycemic load

The glycemic index (GI) is a value assigned to foods based on the speed at which they cause increases in blood glucose levels. [7]

Foods low on the glycemic index release glucose at a slower and more even rate. Foods high on the glycemic index release glucose at a much faster rate.

Low GI foods tend to assist with fat loss, while high GI foods will release energy for recovery after exercise, so one is not better, just used differently.

The more even release of glucose in low glycemic foods is particularly useful in keeping blood glucose under control, but to understand the complete effect a food has on blood sugar, you need to understand how quickly the food causes glucose to enter the bloodstream, as well as how much glucose it will deliver.

Glycemic load does that.

Watermelon, for example, has a high glycemic index (80). But a serving of watermelon has so little carbohydrate (6 g) that the glycemic load is only 5.

A glycemic load of 10 or below is considered low; 20 or above is considered high.

You can find out more about where foods stand in glycemic load and glycemic index in the *International tables of glycemic load and glycemic index*.

Conclusion

Foods that have been processed and refined tend to have:

- Higher sugar per ounce/gram
- Higher salt per ounce/gram
- Lower fibre per ounce/gram
- Lower minerals per ounce/gram
- Lower vitamins per ounce/gram

So, while 2,000 kcal from processed foods has the same, or very similar impact on our total weight as 2,000 kcal from nutrient-rich, fibre-dense foods, the outcome will be very different:

- Higher risk of most diseases
- Higher percentage of body fat
- Lower percentage of muscle mass
- Increased hunger
- Decreased satiety
- Less energy
- Less motivation

Nearly every diet, from low fat to ketogenic, universally agrees that the calories we consume from highly processed foods are not as good for us as the calories within whole foods.

For weight loss, there is calories. For everything else, there is food quality.

If overall weight, and even fat loss, is your goal, your starting point must be calorie balance, but this remains an incomplete picture.

Not considering food quality will impact why you are eating too much, your motivation as well as energy levels.

Quality calories will increase energy, improve mental state and build muscle tissue while reducing total levels of fat and overall chance of disease.

Low quality calories, from processed sources will have almost the exact opposite effect.

Do not, however, make the mistake of thinking that every food you eat must be nutrient dense and whole, because while theoretically this is healthy, it can be a dangerous line of thinking.

Clean eating is a concept that suggests some foods are 'dirty', when they are not.

Banning foods because they are dirty, with little or no nutrient quality or health benefits will simply cause us to overeat them when the dam of will power finally breaks.

Let's face it, some people like things a little dirty!

All diets should have a predominance of healthy foods, and the higher the healthy food ratio, the better the overall health and outcomes, but beyond this you can decide how much of your diet should be nutrient dense whole foods, and how much of your diet should be foods you eat, for no better reason than you enjoy them.

And no more justification is needed than that.

Is a calorie a calorie recap

Key points:

- Not all calories are created equal.
- Some calories make you feel full by filling the digestive tract.
- Protein has a higher thermic effect than other macronutrients.
- No dietary protocol promotes a high ratio of processed and refined foods.
- A higher percentage of calories from processed foods are absorbed.
- Processed foods have less fibre, vitamins and minerals.
- A minimum of 70% of foods should be whole foods.

Things to do:

- Consider your goals and personal preferences.
- Decide on a healthy food ratio that works best for you.
- Listen to your body and be flexible with your ratios over time.

Transform for Life – The Blueprint will help you get the right healthy food ratio for you.

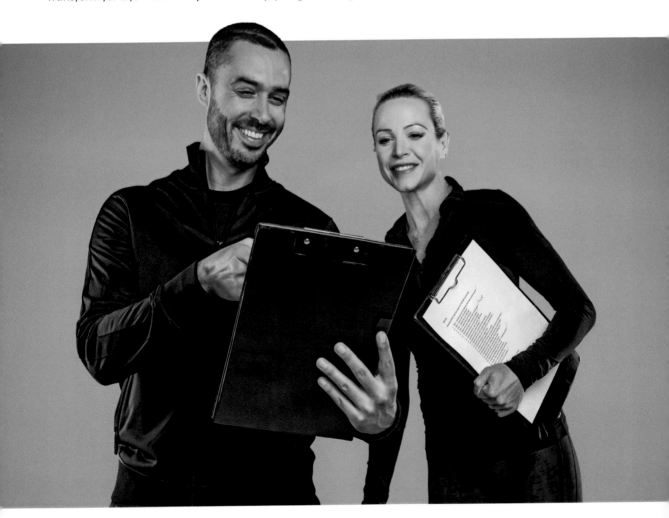

UNDERSTANDING EXERCISE

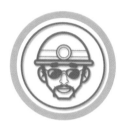

If foods are the building blocks we use to create our body, then exercise is the builder (yes, Rob) we use to shape it and decide how these building blocks are used.

All movement is exercise. Walking the dog, standing up from the couch, running for the bus and even lifting your mug to your lips is exercise.

Below is a simple reminder of the role of calories versus other factors:

Weight loss =	Body composition (fat loss and muscle) =
Amount of calories burned	**Type** of exercise undertaken
Amount of calories consumed	**Type** of calories consumed

Focused exercise such as resistance training and HIIT training is important because:

A.   **Body composition**: Lifting weights and working hard with cardio requires a more muscular and lean physique than just walking. The body adapts and evolves based on relevant stimuli. [1]

B.   **The requirement for balance**: An intelligent workout plan reduces imbalances and potential for injuries.

C.   **Accelerated calorie burn**: We achieve more in a shorter amount of time. [2]

Understanding how to get the most from exercise and what exercise to do will maximise both the effectiveness and speed of evolution your body will experience.

Compliance, compliance, compliance

Whether you decide to exercise for 25 minutes a day six times a week, or 45 minutes a day six times a week should be based on your capacity to maintain rather than your desire for results.

Consistency is always the most important aspect of long-term results, so creating long-term sustainable habits should always drive your decisions.

Any training routine is 100% better than no training routine.

Exercise type ratios

Exercise ratios have so many permeations it is impossible to say what the correct balance is, but if we start from a good point, we can work backwards based on personal goals.

The following recommendation is an approximate balance and roughly what the majority of our workout plans are based on.

- 35% resistance workouts (including circuit-based dumb-bell resistance within PT (cardio and resistance circuit) and bodyweight resistance such as squats, lunges and presses included in some cardio workouts).
- 45% cardio (including HIIT, steady cardio, boxing).
- 20% mobilization/Pilates/active recovery.

As a rough guide, in a 6-workout week this would be:

- 2 x absolute cardio workouts.
- 2 x cardio/resistance hybrid workouts.
- 1 x resistance dominant workout.
- 1 x mobilization/Pilates workout.

Let's take a look at the different training types, why we do them, and when we should do more of them.

Note: *While ratios can change based on goals and preferences, we always recommend participation in all exercise types.*

Why exercise for weight loss?

If creating calorie deficits along with good macronutrient ratios and healthy foods are the key factor for fat loss, why bother exercising?

Heart rate raising exercise is essential for optimal fat loss/muscle repair. [3]

Not specifically cardio, resistance, swimming, running or any other method but any exercise that raises the heart rate.

Exercise creates an environment for our body to utilize protein substrates to rebuild muscle tissue and convert stored fat into energy for use.

1. ALL exercise provides sufficient stimulus to encourage this state.
2. Without surplus calories for a 'muscle building' environment, the additional 'muscle building' benefits of resistance training are less important.
3. With exercise as the key driver of creating a fat-burning and muscle-repairing environment, and both resistance AND cardio providing sufficient physiological stimulus to support this, the choice of which should be done more to lose fat/weight should be based on other factors.

If we neglect exercise in a calorie deficit, we will not stimulate the metabolic process of tissue repair and fat mobilization, therefore any weight loss will almost certainly be a higher percentage of muscle. [4, 5]

This is why exercise is so important.

Lily's Laws 9

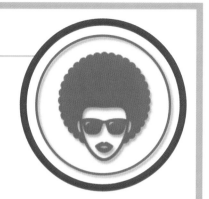

Good news! Lily just found a **NEW** universal law of change.

- Calorie balance
- Anabolic and catabolic flux
- Sufficient carbohydrates
- Sufficient protein
- Sufficient fat
- Drink enough water
- Eat plenty of vegetables
- Limit processed food intake
- **Exercise to stimulate muscle growth and fat loss**

Why cardio training?

Klong

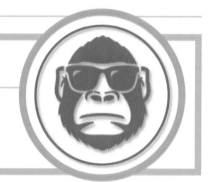

Klong loves it when you do cardio.

You deplete glucose, setting him free from his cage to go on a fat-smashing frenzy!

Why is it that people looking to lose fat require a higher proportion of cardio?

Calories burned

Cardio, especially HIIT or interval training, burns more calories than resistance training.

While burning calories should never be the reason for exercise (food intake and even NEAT – see *The Importance of NEAT* – will invariably be the most important aspects of a calorie deficit) as a choice of training based around an ultimate desire to create an overall calorie reduction, cardio always wins. [6]

Resistance versus Cardio for weight loss

	Duration	No. of workouts	Workout kcal	Weekly kcal	Annual* kcal	Annual weight loss**
Resistance training	45 minutes	6	291	1,750	84,000	24 lb (11 kg)
Cardio training	45 minutes	6	416	2,500	120,000	34 lb (15 kg)
Difference						10 lb (4.5 kg)

*48 weeks training per year.

**3,500 kcal = 1 lb (0.45kg) in body weight. This is a slightly dated calculation, but is used to provide indicative values.

The chart explains the initial reason cardio deserves a slightly higher ratio than resistance training when weight and fat loss is the goal.

This is not suggesting cardio is better than resistance, because it is not. Resistance training has significant long-term benefits around metabolism, muscle definition and strength.

Note: *In a caloric surplus, resistance training deserves a higher ratio for its muscle building qualities and whenever we flux our calories we should take this factor into account and increase our resistance training ratio.*

Other factors

There are three reasons cardio leads our recommended ratios, extending beyond aesthetics:

1. **Cardio equates to a longer, healthier life**. Cardio gives you the heart, lung, hormonal and circulatory benefits that improve and lengthen your life. [7]
2. **Cardio is the queen of compliance**. The endorphins and other feel-good hormones you release keep you coming back. [8]
3. **Cardio and mental health**. Cardio is proven to have a significant positive effect on depression, anxiety and other mental health conditions. [9]

Increase cardio training ratios if:

- You want to lose fat as your primary goal.
- You want to increase lung capacity.
- You want to release endorphins.
- You prefer cardio training (compliance, compliance, compliance!).

Why resistance training?

When we place sufficient tension through muscle fibres to break them down, the body will repair and rebuild them in a process called adaptation.

Resistance training forces our body into this state.

Resistance training with good form also increases bone density and helps prevent osteoporosis as well as increasing our baseline metabolic rate. [10]

Increase resistance training ratios if:

- You want to build muscle.
- You want a stronger metabolism.
- You want to change your body shape.
- You have a specific area of your body you want to work on.
- You want to improve your posture.
- You prefer resistance training (compliance, compliance, compliance!).

Note 1: *While you can increase resistance training ratios, we would never recommend entirely replacing cardio or mobilization.*

Note 2: *Any time you increase your resistance training significantly, you should increase protein intake.*

You can learn more about resistance training in our *Exercise Handbook*, by visiting the following link:

www.teambodyproject.com/additional-resources/

Why mobilization workouts?

Mobilization type workouts have a far different role to play in your overall health in that they support all other types of exercise and daily activities by improving:

- Core stability
- Posture
- Muscle engagement
- Mobility
- Flexibility

People who take part in mobilization workouts are more likely to stay free from injury and improve performance in all other workout types.

Mobilization is the ultimate long-term gain exercise type.

Nobody who has ever followed a mobilization plan has regretted it.

Increase mobilization training ratios if:

- You want to improve posture.
- You want to improve flexibility.
- You want to increase mobility (strength through a range of motion).
- You want to develop better core strength.
- **You prefer mobilization training** (compliance, compliance, compliance!).

Training intelligence

Workouts do not change your body, you do. Workouts are the map you need to follow to reach your destination.

While 'just' working out will achieve good results, developing training intelligence will speed up and even transform your outcomes within the same time frame.

An intelligent approach to exercise will have a significant impact on the results you achieve.

1. Quantity and quality of muscle tissue.
2. Increase or decrease calories burned and fat utilized.
3. Widen range of motion and minimize injuries.

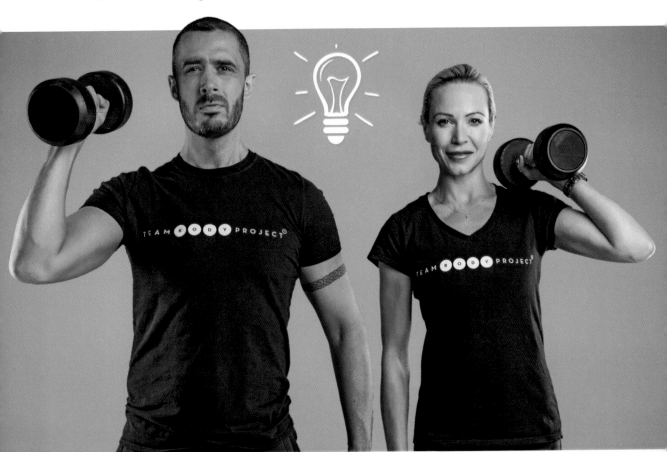

Intensity

Let's take a look at the overall intensity we can apply to any workout.

Intensity levels

1. Going through the motions (LOW effort)

Turning up, completing the movements (with use of gravity and safe momentum) and getting it done. Going through the motions is a fine way to train some of the time, certainly in the early part of your exercise journey.

Compliance is the leading predictor of results, making turning up more important than anything else within this manual.

For all the science and precision, turning up every day is the number one predictor of long-term success.

2. Doing it! (MEDIUM effort)

You're not taking it easy, but you're not taking it to the limit either. This is where most of your workouts will probably be.

3. Taking it to the limit (HIGH effort)

This is the effort given when you push everything off the scale, out of the park. Every pain barrier is breached with every rep, and every set drained and executed for every last ounce of benefit.

Intensity is the overall effort you put into a workout.

Not every workout should be completed at level 3. In fact, this would be considered a bad rather than a good thing. Intelligence is the balance between intensity levels.

Tension

Tension drives results with resistance training.

Set quantities, rep speeds, weights (or load) and total reps are designed to vary, increase, decrease and influence the type of tension your muscles experience.

Without placing muscles under tension, you are just moving your muscles and ligaments around the joint. This is great for mobilization and activation, but if you want to improve the tone, strength or shape of your muscles you will need to force adaptation by applying tension to break the muscles down. [11]

Continuous tension overloads the working muscles and forces the body to adapt.

Rob

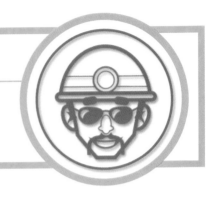

When muscle is broken down, Rob comes and builds it back stronger and better. If it's not broken, Rob won't fix it!

So break it!

Muscular engagement

During resistance workouts you must learn to keep your muscles under tension through both the concentric (against gravity) and more importantly eccentric (with gravity) part of the movement.

Think of a press up.

By bending your elbows and going towards the ground you are being assisted by gravity, meaning this part of the movement could actually happen with no effort. You could literally fall through the eccentric part of the movement with gravity assisting you.

Slowing this movement down by controlling and engaging the muscle to work against gravity is imperative for best results.

We call this eccentric control. You can either engage your muscles to fight against gravity through the movement to generate results or you can allow gravity to do the work for you and give the eccentric half of your resistance results away.

The drive up against gravity (concentric) requires muscular effort, so there is always a forced contraction, but an additional focus on muscle engagement remains important to maximize engagement and tension and minimize momentum.

Important: Whenever you are confused which part of the movement is concentric and which part of the movement is eccentric, simply consider which part of the movement is against gravity and which part is with it.

Understanding how to use your muscles correctly during movements, how to dial up intensity on cardio and how to move between effort levels, combine to create training intelligence.

Once you have developed training intelligence, every workout, regardless of difficulty level, changes depending on how you approach it.

Example:

On a day when you are feeling a little fatigued you have a few options:

- A high level workout at 1 – **low effort**
- A medium level workout at 2 – **medium effort**
- A low level workout at 3 – **high effort**

I find the least personal benefit and sense of satisfaction from choosing a high level workout at effort level 1 and the most benefit from a low level workout executed at level 3, but every choice has a place.

On the other end of the scale, never underestimate the benefits of a level 1 or 2 workout completed with excellent muscle control and tension with level 3 effort.

Of course, the most difficult workout would be high level with level 3 effort, but developing the intelligence to understand what the intention behind the workout is on any given day will produce more diverse and enjoyable results.

Rest and active recovery

How long should I exercise per week?

As a guideline, between 150 minutes (20 minutes per day) and 450 minutes (60 minutes per day) of focused exercise per week is recommended.

Twenty minutes of exercise a day is sufficient to change your physiological environment to a fat burning/muscle building one. This is why we can expect great results from shorter durations of exercise.

So what is the difference between exercising for 20 minutes and 45 minutes?

1. **Calories**. The less you exercise you do, the more consideration you have to give to the amount of food you consume.
2. **Progress**. Your fitness levels, strength and other benefits will not happen as quickly.
3. **Speed of fat loss**. Since the body has less exercise-induced muscle damage, it also has less need for protein substrates and therefore less need to mobilize fat as a fuel resource.

What if you decide to exercise for MORE than 450 minutes a week (around 60 minutes a day)?

At up to 60 minutes per day you will be in a more consistently positive metabolic environment, with a higher calorie burn and a good speed of both progress and fat loss.

However, your body has a limit (that will vary from person to person) on the amount of protein it can synthesize for repair and the amount of fat it can mobilize for energy per week.

For this reason, beyond 60 minutes of exercise, you will experience negligible gains, and would require additional calories in order to support your additional training without losing muscle.

Unless you have specific performance goals, like training for a marathon or competing in sport, training beyond 450 minutes per week will simply increase your food bill and increase your risk of overtraining.

Exercise spread

We have a preference for your total exercise being spread over the week, based on two factors:

1. The psychological habit benefits of daily training.
2. The physiological metabolic benefits of daily training (fat burning/muscle building environment).

Training for 90 minutes twice a week is great if it fits your lifestyle, but it falls short on the above points when compared to 30 minutes, five times a week.

Active recovery versus sedentary recovery

Some people do very well on sedentary rest whereas others thrive on active rest.

Active rest is any gentle exercise-based activity on a rest day. Some people find the physiological benefits of active rest are more positive than sedentary rest, alongside experiencing the psychological benefit of doing something.

A light swim, a meandering bike ride, a gentle workout or a brisk walk would be good examples.

Sedentary rest should be self explanatory. Put your feet up for a well-earned break! Just as many, if not more people find the physiological and psychological benefits of total rest to be greater than active rest.

There is no difference in long-term results, regardless of the type of rest you choose, so choice should be driven by compliance and personal preference.

What we strongly recommend against is no rest. In any given seven day period a minimum of one day should not include intensive exercise.

Note: *Active rest should NOT be calculated in your total exercise time.*

Longer planned rests

Having a week or two off for total rest a couple of times a year is fine, provided compliance is returned to, but equally there is no specific benefit to having long breaks from movement-based activity.

While extended total rest from exercise has no specific benefits, it is important to take your foot off the gas every couple of months with a period of less challenging workouts.

You cannot keep pushing your body, week after week, and expect it to continue making progress.

We recommend a week of lighter exercise every 6-8 weeks to prepare your body for the planned progress ahead.

These lighter periods will also help you avoid forced rests through overtraining or injury.

Understanding exercise recap

Key points:

- Exercise is essential for fat burning and muscle building.
- Cardio burns the most calories and also offers other health benefits.
- Resistance encourages muscle growth and superior repair.
- Mobilization reduces injuries and improves performance.
- Training intelligence – intensity and time under tension improve results.
- Planned rest times are important.

Things to do:

- Decide on an exercise plan that supports your goals.
- Practise the tension and intensity principles.
- Build in rest times.

Transform for Life – The Blueprint will help you choose the right exercise programme for your fitness levels and goals.

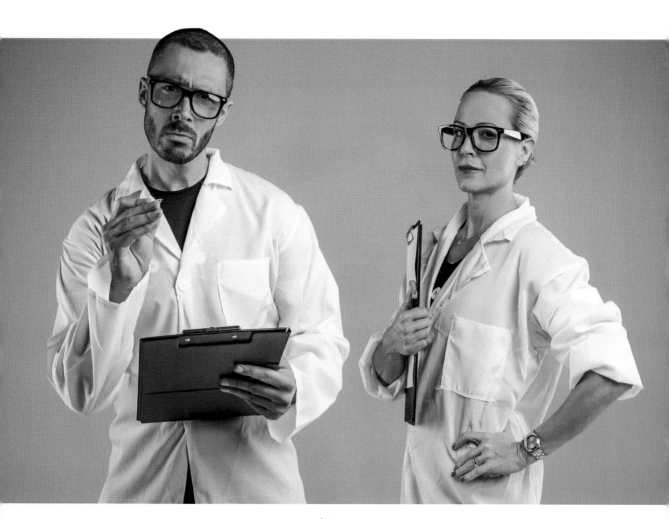

THE IMPORTANCE OF NEAT

Non-Exercise Activity Thermogenesis (NEAT) is activity beyond your focused exercise and natural metabolism. It's a combination of your normal daily activity, your posture and your general movement – anything that uses energy beyond deliberate exercise and your baseline metabolic rate (BMR).

While people do have BMR differences, research indicates that the variance in resting metabolic rate from person to person is small (up to 300 kcal between the fastest and slowest metabolisms in people of similar height and weight and without thyroid conditions).[1]

On the other hand, research shows the difference in NEAT is estimated to be between 200 and 500 kcal and even as high as 2,000 kcal in exceptional circumstances.

NEAT matters a lot. How many steps you walk, what you do when the adverts come on the telly, whether you take the stairs or the lift, how you fill your break times at work, what activities you do with the kids, how much you fidget, what you do when your train is running late.

If you're trying to lose weight, NEAT could be factored in as an essential part of your daily activity. NEAT is not spontaneous in the majority of the population, it needs to be planned like everything else.

An extra 250 kcal from NEAT alongside an extra 250 kcal from your work out means you have burned an additional 500 kcal. That's 3,500 kcal a week, which could equates to around 1 lb of body weight.

To improve your NEAT:

- Buy a tracker
- Make good choices
- Be active

Moderate versus Low NEAT over 12 weeks:

	Person 1	Person 2
NEAT	Moderate NEAT +500 kcal per day	Low NEAT +250 kcal per day
Calorie intake	1,500 kcal	1,500 kcal
Exercise	30 minutes = 250 kcal	30 minutes = 250 kcal
Weekly difference	1,750 more burned	1,750 less burned
12 week weight difference	Lost 6 lb (3 kg) more than person 2*	Lost 6 lb (3 kg) less than person 1*

*assuming 3,500 kcal = 1 lb in body weight

The difference between a low and a moderate level of NEAT over 12 weeks was 21,000 kcal.

In terms of food that would be:

- 50 cheeseburgers (400 kcal)
- 100 bags of potato chips (210 kcal)
- 400 slices of bread (52 kcal)

In terms of exercise it would be:

- 84 cardio workouts (30 minute sessions)
- 150 Pilates workouts (30 minute sessions)

NEAT is a very important aspect of your overall health plan that can make the difference between long-term success and long-term struggle.

Factor it in!

Subconscious NEAT

A seldom discussed but crucial factor in weight management is the different effects higher and lower food consumption has on certain body types/people and NEAT*. [2]

Ectomorphs – Ectomorphs have smaller bone structures and longer limbs. The increased 'speed' of an ectomorph's metabolism is less to do with BMR and more closely linked with increased NEAT. An ectomorph may often struggle to gain weight because they subconsciously 'move more' when they eat more calories. While it may seem that an ectomorph has a faster metabolism, often what they have is an insatiable need to burn what they consume.

Endomorphs – Endomorphs have a larger bone structure, with shorter limbs. This body type is considered by some to have higher propensity to gain weight.

Additional calories consumed do not result in an additional 'need' to burn off calories, making weight gain common. Furthermore, when fewer calories are consumed, endomorphs may subconsciously 'move less'. Creating the false belief that the metabolism is too slow.

This is why tracking NEAT is so important.

Ectomorphs (or some people) = Eat more, move more. Eat less, move the same.
Endomorphs (or some people) = Eat less, move less. Eat more, move the same.

Visit pages 179-80 in *The Blueprint* for more information on body types.

Body types is a somewhat controversial area. There are understandable points of contention around whether the body type itself is a relevant factor in influencing subconscious NEAT (or anything else for that matter).

However, there is no doubt that subconscious NEAT itself is an important factor, regardless of your body type and whether this influences your choices - NEAT must always be factored in.

Lily's Laws 10

Good news! Lily just found a NEW universal law of change.

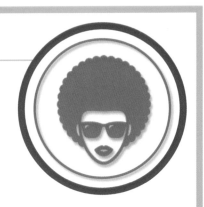

- Calorie balance
- Anabolic and catabolic flux
- Sufficient carbohydrates
- Sufficient protein
- Sufficient fat
- Drink enough water
- Eat plenty of vegetables
- Limit processed food intake
- Exercise to stimulate muscle growth and fat loss
- **NEAT is an important aspect of your metabolic rate**

The importance of NEAT recap

Key points:

- NEAT is the activity we do beyond focused exercise.
- It is not catabolic so can be increased with confidence.

Things to do:

- Buy or download a tracker.
- Find out how much NEAT you do.
- Increase levels to help you achieve a calorie deficit.

Transform for Life – The Blueprint will help you choose the right amount of NEAT.

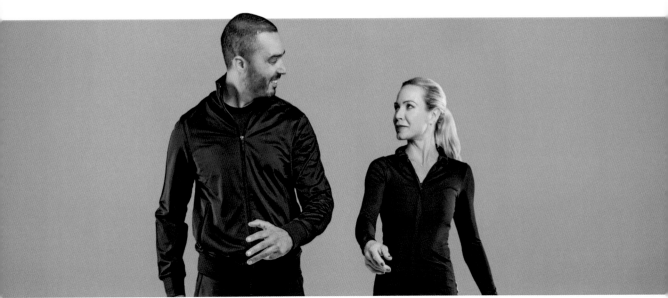

POPULAR DIETS

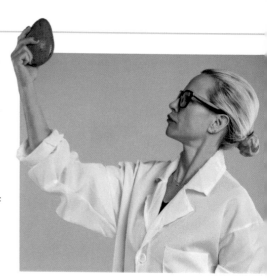

Every year, it seems there is a new popular diet that everybody is trying.

Rule 1 of nutrition: If a diet is in fashion, probably don't follow it.

What looks stylish today, looks dated tomorrow. The classics stay around for the long haul, which is why I can still wear my flares.

The nutrition classics of macronutrient balance, calorie control, plenty of vegetables and limiting processed foods never go out of fashion.

That is not to say that popular diets can't be effective, but if you are going to follow one, do so with your eyes open.

Clean eating

A few years ago, a number of celebrities and fitness professionals put their weight behind a concept that became known as clean eating.[1]

This concept was paired heavily with the idea of superfoods – foods with a higher than average nutrient density – and the idea that sugar was responsible for pretty much everything, from weight gain to global warming and rising taxes.

What is clean eating?

Clean eating is the consumption of foods that are whole and unprocessed. An easy way of identifying a clean food is checking if it fits into one of the following categories:

- It flew (like a bird)
- It ran (like a pig or chicken)
- It swam (like a fish)
- It fell or was picked (like an apple or a coconut)
- It grew (like a potato or a turnip)

Most will consider that grains, like rice, oats and quinoa are clean but some will not. Overall the closer to the original state the food is, the cleaner it is.

Example: unprocessed meats like chicken breast, are considered to be cleaner than processed ones, like chorizo.

Dirty foods would be foods that have been processed or refined in any way. The more refined or processed they are, the dirtier they are.

Note: *I know, I know, 'dirty' foods sound so naughty and exciting.*

These include:

- Most breakfast cereals
- White bread, pasta and rice
- Confectionary
- Processed meats
- Pastries, potato chips and cookies

Of course, any sensible person will tell you that no food is dirty and no food is clean. Some foods have higher fibre, less sugar and more nutrients. Some foods support our health and some foods, eaten in large amounts, can be damaging to our health.

They aren't clean or dirty, although a part of me wishes they were.

Benefits of clean eating

When viewed in the context of weight loss and transformative health, clean eating offers a few specific benefits if it can be adhered to:

- High fibre content
- High nutrient value
- Lower requirement for tracking due to superior hunger signalling, low calorie density and increased fibre content

The most interesting of these is the lower requirement for tracking. In my experience, those who adhere to a 100% clean eating protocol have less need for tracking than those who do not. They do, however, still need to take baths. Clean eating does not extend to overall hygiene.

Should I follow clean eating?

A diet that is high in trans fats, sugars and salt and low in fibre and nutrients is bad news for your health and weight, which is why any sensible dietician or nutritionist recommends a predominance of calories from healthy sources.

While there are proven health benefits to ensuring a minimum of 70% of food comes from healthy sources, there is no evidence to suggest that complete elimination of dirty foods creates additional benefits.

People who have no interest or desire to eat processed foods or drink alcohol and do not wish to spend any time tracking intake can consider clean eating as a solution to weight management.

In my experience, there are very few people who would find this to be practical or desirable.

It is better to take all food into account and create a health plan based around eating a predominance of healthy foods in context with your goals, emotional eating habits and tastes.

Benefits of clean eating

- Very healthy
- Tracking becomes less important

Problems with clean eating

- Can cause an unhealthy relationship with food
- Difficult to maintain for most people

Important: Is sugar addictive?

The science on sugar has historically been clear.

Sugar does not have the *physiological* addictive properties of cocaine, nicotine or alcohol, nor does it have the severe withdrawal symptoms that would be experienced when refraining from these substances. [2]

On the other hand, I have witnessed sugar to have stronger *psychologically* addictive qualities than almost anything else. Some people have an overwhelming dependency on sugar to numb emotions, cope with difficult situations or change the way they feel.

On top of this, neuroscientists have recently shown that sugar leads to the release of dopamine and overconsumption leads to tolerance so increasingly large levels are required to experience the same dopamine effect. This would seem to mimic some of the hallmarks of drug addiction.[3]

It is understandable that those who consider themselves 'sugar addicts' often see the best solution to avoid it at all costs.

The problem with this ultimate solution is that it has a less than 1% long-term success rate as any reintroduction of sugar to the diet is perceived as failure and triggers uncontrollable rates of consumption.

My personal challenge has historically been sugar. I would spend months abstaining from sugar, only to succumb to outrageous binges the moment a tiny morsel of sugar passed my lips, playing 'With or Without You' on full volume to let the sugar know exactly how I felt about our relationship.

Despite some substantial evidence to the contrary, I felt convinced it was physiological and I was addicted it.

Breaking the negative sugar cycle

Certain foods with sugar in them taste really good. There is nothing wrong with eating food for reasons that extend no further than enjoyment of taste. Refined sugar has no nutritional benefits that cannot be obtained from healthier sources, but that does not mean it shouldn't be consumed, simply that it shouldn't be consumed in excess.

Getting caught up in whether it is or isn't a physiological addiction is not particularly useful, so we need to look towards the information that can support us in change.

1.   **Less than 1% of people successfully live without sugar for the rest of their lives.**

Very few people will successfully abstain from sugar for life. If we seek this route we set ourselves up for failure. Therefore, declaring ourselves to be physiological addicts that must abstain entirely has no benefit regardless of whether it is true.

2.   **Many people who perceive themselves as sugar addicts are eating reasonable levels of sugar within a healthy diet.**

I can include myself in that statistic. I have witnessed many thousands of people successfully break the sugar cycle. Whether they were caught by psychological or physiological addiction is far less relevant than whether they can break it.

And they can.

How to break the sugar cycle

If you are a sugar addict, the greatest challenge you will have in your diet will be eating sensible amounts of it.

The longer you live without sugar, the greater the propensity for uncontrollable rebound consumption.

This proven system has been used to break the sugar cycle many times:

1. A short period of total abstinence

You won't be surprised to learn that total elimination in the long-term is a bad idea, but short-term abstinence to reset tolerance, insulin levels and take control of the sharp end of emotional eating habits is beneficial. This can last anywhere between two and six weeks.

2. Reintroduction of sugar

When you feel ready, it's time to take consideration of foods you want to consume in the longer-term and introduce them in smaller quantities and at times you decide you will eat them.

Many people are frightened of reintroducing sugar, but if the reintroduction is not planned and prepared for, one of two things will happen:

Emotional reintroduction

Sugar gets reintroduced to the diet in an emotional way and the pattern of emotional consumption of sugar resumes.

Relaxed reintroduction

Sugar gets reintroduced at a time when you are relaxed and unprepared for the dopamine. You roll back into Binge Town.

By reintroducing sugar to your diet on **your** terms, you are reshaping your relationship with sugar and teaching yourself that you can have healthy amounts.

3. Letting go of isolated incidents

Some people experience isolated incidents when they binge on sugar the same way some people come home after a very difficult day and drink a bottle of wine. This does not make them alcoholics.

Having an incident does not make you an addict, it makes you human and vulnerable to the ups and downs of life in the same way as everybody else. If this happens it is not important. What is important is that you do not allow sugar binges to become habits.

By following this plan, over time you will develop a healthy relationship with sugar that is directly in line with your personal long-term goals.

Vegan

What is Vegan?

A vegan diet is the exclusion of all animal products, including cheese and eggs. This has become an increasingly popular dietary approach in the last few years.

My wife, Alexandra, is vegan. I would like to be vegan but struggle without any animal products, so instead consume as few as I can. I eat fish twice a week and eggs twice a week.

I am a vegan who eats fish. And eggs. This actually makes me not vegan. Don't tell anybody!

We do not claim that a vegan diet is the best diet for health. Although there are benefits, which we will discuss below, there are challenges too. With a few observational exceptions linked to certain types of cancers and other diseases, there are no benefits you can get from a vegan diet that you cannot get from an alternative diet. We choose to eat vegan (yes, yes I know, I'm not vegan) because we believe it is possible to eat a healthy diet without animal products and this is important to us, ethically.

Our personal choice and preference towards being vegan has nothing to do with overall health and we certainly don't fly around the world, emitting large amounts of carbon into the atmosphere, explaining to people that eating vegan is better for the environment.

Benefits of eating vegan

A good vegan diet, especially one that is high in plant-based foods, scores very well on satiety factors, as vegetables and fruits especially are voluminous and take up plenty of space in the digestive tract.

Vegan foods are also packed full of nutrients, vitamins and minerals, scoring very highly on nutrient density. I have found that many vegans struggle to eat enough calories, which could be seen as a benefit in the short-term (and a problem in the long-term – what do you reckon, Rob?).

The potential health benefits of vegan diets are exciting, including reported observational improvements around heart health, reduced cancer risks, improved kidney function and reduced chances of Alzheimer's. [4,5]

As current studies have been observational, conclusive studies to confirm that a vegan diet is causing these effects simply don't exist. There is no way of knowing if it is other lifestyle factors that vegans share, such as being more likely to exercise or less likely to eat high levels of processed foods, smoke or drink alcohol, that are behind these benefits. Regardless, a good vegan diet is an excellent choice from an overall health perspective, and provided protein is consumed correctly and supplementation is considered for any potential deficiencies, this is a diet that can help you lose weight and be healthy.

Problems with eating vegan

A good vegan diet needs to be carefully planned and considered. Poorly planned vegan diets often present with nutrient deficiencies. People who succeed with a vegan lifestyle in the long-term have a solid understanding of the diet and how to ensure it works for them. This diet is not a magic bullet.

Vegans can be more at risk of having low levels of vitamin D, vitamin B12, omega 3s, iron, calcium and zinc, although most of this would be associated with poor quality vegan foods. A vegan diet is only good if you eat high quality vegan foods. If you eat a predominance of junk vegan foods it is every bit as bad as any other diet and a poorly planned vegan diet can be very bad indeed.

The heart benefits, reduced cancer risks and other benefits are associated with eating high nutrient foods in exactly the same way a non-vegan diet is. In most instances vitamin B12, D vitamins and omega 3s are recommended to supplement a vegan diet.

Should I follow a vegan diet?

There is no strong reason you shouldn't, but on the other hand there is no strong reason you should. The overall health benefits of a good vegan diet stem from the same key points that all healthy protocols share.

Lily's Laws

Lily wants to remind you of the universal laws of change.

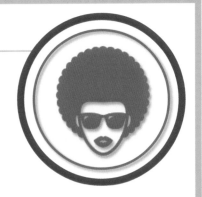

- Calorie balance
- Anabolic and catabolic flux
- Sufficient carbohydrates
- Sufficient protein
- Sufficient fat
- Drink enough water
- Eat plenty of vegetables
- Limit processed food intake
- Exercise to stimulate muscle growth and fat loss
- NEAT is an important aspect of your metabolic rate

If you don't like meat, fish or animal products or find it important for you ethically not to eat animal products this is an excellent diet to follow.

If you love eating animal products, this is a dreadful diet. For you.

Benefits of eating vegan

- Plenty of promises around reducing disease.
- Low energy density/high nutrient density.
- Animal welfare and environmental benefits.

Problems with eating vegan

- Can be as bad as any other diet.
- Needs work to get it right.
- Can cause deficiencies very easily.

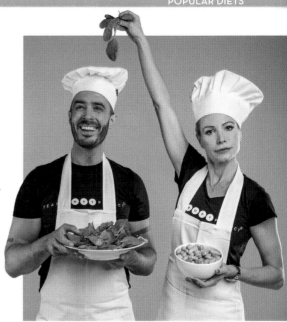

The ketogenic diet

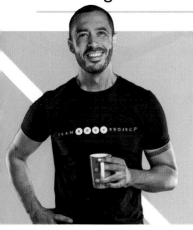

The Kettle-genic diet

The Ketogenic diet is not to be confused with the Kettle-genic diet, a popular diet in Great Britain on building sites, industrial estates and offices.

Those following the Kettle-genic diet insist on having the kettle on at all times, drinking eight or more cups of tea a day. This harmful fad diet can potentially cause excess biscuit consumption.

What is it?

A ketogenic diet is a diet that places the body into a state called ketosis, whereby fats are burned instead of carbohydrates for use as energy. A ketogenic diet requires the consumption of high amounts of fat, adequate amounts of protein, and very low amounts of carbohydrates.

Important note: *A ketogenic diet is not the same as a high-protein diet, where un-utilized protein can go through a process called gluconeogenesis, converting protein to glucose and preventing ketosis.* [6]

How it works?

Once the body is depleted of stored glucose and glycogen, it transports fat into the liver and produces ketones that can be used for energy, even for tasks that would normally be the preserve of carbohydrates, like brain function.

There is usually a difficult period in this diet prior to the body releasing ketones and after stored glucose and glycogen is depleted. However, once this is broken through, the body will be functioning perfectly well in the absence of insulin and glucose.

A high level of circulating glucagon and low levels of insulin make this diet very effective at targeting fat stores for energy.

From a simple weight-loss perspective a ketogenic diet is very effective.

Note: *If you are going to follow a ketogenic diet, do it properly.* **You must eat at least 70% fat.**

Problems with eating a ketogenic diet

The ketogenic diet promises faster fat loss results than most other diets, but there are drawbacks.

At least 95% of people cannot sustain this diet in the long-term.

You may be one of the 5%, and for this reason I would never suggest that you shouldn't try it. If you decide to, please do seek alternative advice from your doctor or a dietician to check you have no conditions that would contraindicate it.

This diet is NOT advised within *Transform for Life* **recommendations.**

The science on whether or not a ketogenic diet can work in the long-term seems to be getting stronger. Followers will insist it is great, where opponents will insist it is harmful, but again, we need to look beyond the science and towards the compliance.

1. **Sustainability**: Most people cannot follow this diet in the long-term.
2. **Restrictive**: It seriously limits choice.
3. **Performance**: High-intensity workouts become much harder.
4. **Muscle growth**: Protein synthesis in the absence of insulin is much slower.

Conclusion

The ketogenic diet stands in direct opposition to some of our recommendations, but it can be effective. However, for most people, there are more balanced ways of achieving long-term results. [7]

When people ask if a ketogenic diet can work, my answer is usually yes, but there is almost certainly a more sustainable, individual and balanced way for you to approach transformative nutrition. Most diets are successful for the same reasons.

Lily's Laws

Lily won't let go of this now!

- Calorie balance
- Anabolic and catabolic flux
- Sufficient carbohydrates
- Sufficient protein
- Sufficient fat
- Drink enough water
- Eat plenty of vegetables
- Limit processed food intake
- Exercise to stimulate muscle growth and fat loss
- NEAT is an important aspect of your metabolic rate

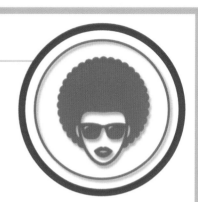

Benefits of the ketogenic diet

- Promotes fat loss
- Can be positive for those with insulin sensitivity and sugar 'addiction'
- Often removes large amounts of processed foods by default

Problems with the ketogenic diet

- Poor performance
- Low compliance
- Highly restrictive
- Poor muscle growth

Intermittent fasting

What is intermittent fasting?

Intermittent fasting is fasting applied intermittently. Yup, it does exactly what it says on the tin.

It is the opposite of the 'little and often' approach since it is more focused on longer periods without food alongside larger portions when we are eating. We could call fasting *more food, less often* but that isn't as marketable as intermittent fasting, so nobody does.

This *more food, less often* approach may be skipping one meal a day, having whole days with no meals or any number of varying durations of 'fast' and 'feast' in between.

There are three main ways people approach fasting:

1. Meal skipping

Skip a predetermined amount of meals in a week with the ultimate goal of eating fewer calories. Example: Skip breakfast every day.

2. Total day fasting

Limit your calories to approximately 500 kcal on fasting days and avoid exercise on these days.

3. Shrink the eating window

Reverse the amount of time in your day to include eight hours of eating time and 16 hours of fasting time (usually paired with specific exercise-led nutrient timing and fasted cardio).

Benefits of intermittent fasting

When fasting, we deplete the body of glucose and stored glycogen within the muscles and start the process of releasing glucagon and freeing fat for energy from stores. [8]

Provided you are not exercising on fasting days this could be positive. If you do exercise on a fasting day, Rob won't have any materials to work with. So it's probably best you don't.

In some ways flux is a less extreme version of the intermittent fasting protocol. Intermittent fasting creates an overall calorie deficit, with the deficit being created in fasting periods, rather than in a more steady way.

For some people this is a more convenient method of creating an overall calorie deficit.

On top of this, there are benefits unique to fasting beyond caloric reduction:

- It teaches discipline.
- You learn hunger management.
- It develops craving control.
- It helps us understand the difference between physical hunger (body hunger) and psychological hunger (appetite), covered in the *Emotional eating guide* (pages 128-137) in *The Art of Change* section.

Problems with intermittent fasting

Despite what some may say, intermittent fasting does not allow you to escape the fundamental rules of health and weight management.

Any suggestion that provided you have fasting days you can eat whatever you want the rest of the time, is not accurate.

There are potential issues with fasting too:

- **Sleep**: Many people report poor sleep on fasting days.
- **Muscle loss**: With such low calorie amounts, the body can start raiding muscle stores to convert to energy (Klong gets bored when he's free for too long).
- **Energy**: Fewer calories means fewer nutrients which can mean less energy.

Some people experience all of the above problems, some experience none. As always, the only way you will know is by trying it yourself.

Compliance is another factor to consider. For some people, staying compliant on fasting days is impossibly hard and this would rule it out immediately.

Conclusion

Net calorie deficit, macronutrient balance, regular exercise and a predominance of high quality food will always remain the priority for health and long-term weight management.

Fasting does not allow us to circumvent the laws of thermodynamics, it simply provides us with a different method of creating calorie balances and imbalances.

The initial choice as to whether intermittent fasting is right for you is best based on the following factors:

- Whether it is easier for you to implement within your lifestyle and circumstances.
- Whether you find it easier to miss meals than count calories or track portions (after a baseline is established).
- Whether you find fasting easier to comply with than other methods of health management.

Positives of fasting

- Teaches good hunger management and craving control.
- Promotes glucagon release and fat loss.
- Can be a simple method of creating a calorie deficit.

Negatives of fasting

- Many people report poor sleep on fasting days.
- With such low calorie amounts, the body can start raiding muscle stores to convert to energy.
- Less calories, means less nutrients which can mean less energy on fasting days.
- For some people, the compliance on fasting days is impossibly hard.

Paleo diet

The Paleo diet is a modern diet requiring the exclusive consumption of foods presumed to have been the only foods consumed by early humans during the Paleolithic era.

Suggested make up of a standard Paleo diet (there are variants):

- 55% of daily calories from seafood and lean meat, evenly divided.
- 15% of daily calories from each of fruits, vegetables, and nuts and seeds.
- No dairy, almost no grains, no added salt, no added sugar.

This diet is usually particularly high in protein, which makes it different from the ketogenic diet, which is high in fat.

Benefits of a Paleo diet

As is consistent with all healthy diets, the main benefits come from an increased amount of vegetables, quality proteins and fats and a reduction in processed foods.

This is a standard theme in many diets and is also true of the Paleo diet, which is simply a brand attached to a way of eating fewer processed foods, higher amounts of vegetables and specifically the elimination of grains which were not available in the Paleolithic era. The benefits of this healthy diet are based on consistent factors, regardless of what it is called.

Problems with the Paleo diet

Knowledge of ratios of animal and plant foods in the diets of early humans is circumstantial and highly debatable, making the theory behind this diet questionable at best. However, the theory behind the diet is somewhat irrelevant as the diet itself is healthy, with similar components to the Mediterranean diet.

There are potential deficiencies in vitamin D and calcium, but this is avoidable with a sensible approach. The main problem with the Paleo diet, like clean eating, is the restriction it places on the participant. Making certain foods contraband creates feelings of guilt based on unsubstantiated evidence suggesting that consumption of grains or any processed foods is responsible for disease. Processed foods usually have lower nutritional density, higher sugar, higher trans-fat and higher sodium levels and this makes them less healthy than non-processed foods. Eating them in high levels is proven to be bad for your health; eating small amounts is not.

Conclusion

The concept behind this diet is based on unsubstantiated evidence but the diet is good.

Is it sensible to increase the amounts of fruits and vegetables and reduce quantities of domesticated grains? On balance, it probably is and for certain autoimmune diseases, such as celiac, it can be a very important dietary change.

Is it sensible to reduce processed foods in our diets? Yes.

Is this the way Paleolithic populations ate? I don't know. I imagine they ate whatever they could get their hands on, including mud, beetles and stinging nettles if they were hungry enough.

Were Paleolithic populations healthier than we are now? I have no idea, but then nor does anybody else.

Once again, if the overall make-up of the Paleo diet suits your palate, lifestyle and goals, there is nothing to suggest it is not a good diet to follow. You can call it whatever you like. Including Paleo. If you want a real caveman diet, I've got a lovely slug and nettle soup on the boil. Provided we don't tell Lily about the 'theory' behind this diet, I'd say she would like it.

Lily's Laws

- Calorie balance
- Anabolic and catabolic flux
- Sufficient carbohydrates
- Sufficient protein
- Sufficient fat
- Drink enough water
- Eat plenty of vegetables
- Limit processed food intake
- Exercise to stimulate muscle growth and fat loss
- NEAT is an important aspect of your metabolic rate

Positives of the Paleo diet

- High protein levels for muscle repair
- Lots of vegetables and fruits
- Limiting on processed foods

Negatives of the Paleo diet

- Highly restrictive

Popular diets conclusion

The YOU diet

If you choose to eat a diet with a predominance of processed foods with an understanding of the associated health consequences, you can do so. Regardless of how many 'bad' foods you are eating, if you control your calorie intake, you can still manage your weight, although managing your body composition will be much trickier.

Conversely, if you choose to eat a diet that eliminates an entire source or type of food, you could do this too. Provided you understand and feel comfortable with any potential consequences that permanent restrictions may produce, there is nothing to suggest this would not be the best method for you.

In my experience, 99% of people find success sits somewhere between these two extremes. Food is not good or bad, clean or dirty. It is just food. Some foods can protect against disease and some foods can contribute to it. Some foods are highly nutritious and some foods are full of trans fats, sugars and sodium.

Transform for Life will help you create a diet that works for you, in line with your goals, your ethics, your preferences and your compliance capabilities.

This is the only diet that matters.

By tracking and measuring how we are responding, both psychologically and physiologically, to foods and exercise, we can adapt accordingly.

The variables – macronutrient ratios, healthy food ratios, calorie quantities, flux ratios, exercise quantity and type – will vary from person to person; there is no right answer.

Find your own Goldilocks zone where your desired results pair with a diet and exercise routine that is both sustainable and enjoyable for you.

This is the YOU diet.

If you want to call it the *'Dirty Diet'* you have my absolute approval.

THE LAWS OF CHANGE

All living organisms must continuously consume and break down food to survive. Food supplements us with the raw materials we need.

While catabolism is constantly breaking down our muscle tissue and fat, anabolism is constantly building new muscle and hopefully, a little less fat.

This never-ending process is the function of our metabolism. It never stops.

In your lifetime you will synthesise around 990 lb (450 kg) of protein.

If you weighed 165 lb (75 kg), that would mean you entirely rebuild yourself, from scratch, six times.

This opens an exciting door of opportunity – through food and exercise you can rebuild your body to be a healthy one.

Yet in the process of getting healthy we become so focused on the breaking down fat that we forget building is an important element too.

The fundamentals we have discovered in these chapters can be applied to our own body to create the personal *Blueprint* for our health. Through these fundamentals we can:

1. Get rid of unwanted, ineffective and unhealthy fat (with Klong).
2. Build healthy, lean muscle tissue (with Rob).
3. Have more energy, feel better and change our lives.

Below I have outlined the fundamentals of change that should be followed to ensure sustainable results.

Then I have outlined the secondary laws of change that while important, can be seen on a sliding scale of application.

Fundamentals of physical change

Law 1: To lose weight you must be in a calorie deficit (hypocaloric)

Whether this deficit is created by fewer calories or more exercise, this law is absolute. If you are not in a deficit, you will not lose weight.

If weight loss is your goal, your blueprint must be built around this concept. Every other law is based around the quality (body composition) and sustainability (compliance and metabolic factors) of your weight loss.

Note: *To gain weight you must be in a calorie surplus (hypercaloric).*

Law 2: Calorie flux; chronic exposure to calorie deficits will compromise anabolic processes

On the one hand, we must have a calorie deficit if we want to lose weight, but on the other hand we need to ensure our body is releasing hormones and has sufficient protein substates to repair and improve healthy tissue. We manage rebuilding within an absolute deficit through calorie flux.

Law 3: Forced adaptation through exercise

Exercise places your body in 'fat burning and muscle building' mode. The body evolves based on stimulus. If you want to lose fat and not muscle, exercise is essential.

Law 4: Food quality and hydration

A predominantly 'healthy' ratio of foods will support your results. Eat plenty of vegetables and stay hydrated.

Try and keep your ratio of healthy food as high as you can while ensuring you are enjoying your meals.

Law 5: Compliance rules them all

If we presented the first four laws to an android, it would achieve entirely predictable results every time. Humans are not so compliant; this is what makes us interesting but also what makes us less predictable.

Every food you eat, every workout you do and every method you implement relies on your ability to be compliant with it in the long-term. The compliance factor permeates through every page of this book and should be infused into your *Blueprint*.

- 95% compliance on an 80% 'good' plan gets incredible results.
- 50% compliance on a 100% 'perfect' plan gets no results.

Be consistent, not perfect.

Weight loss and baseline body composition factors are impacted by primary laws of physical change. Specific results and outcomes are impacted by the secondary laws.

Secondary laws are very important to your physical improvements, but the extent to which they matter is variable and your application of them negotiable.

If you want to have visible abs and a very toned body, you will need to pay closer attention to them than if you want to lose a little weight and live a balanced lifestyle.

When it comes to secondary laws, it is imperative you line up your expectations with your behaviour.

You cannot expect the same results eating 70% healthy foods and exercising for 20 minutes a day as you can when eating 95% healthy foods and exercising for 60 minutes a day.

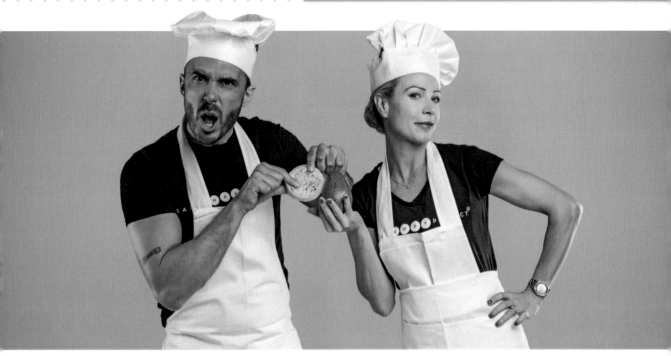

Secondary laws of physical change

Law 1: Macronutrient ratio

You will need a minimum level of protein to ensure muscle retention, especially in a deficit.

Carbohydrate tolerance will be varied and higher ratios could promote fat storage, but support energy and performance.

Higher fat ratios promote glucagon production but could compromise performance.

Your ideal ratio will change over time and depend on your goals. The only way to know which ratio is right for you is to try it.

Law 2: Type and quantity of exercise

A. Cardio will promote a higher calorie burn, putting a larger dent in your deficit (as well as offering heart, lung and emotional benefits).
B. Resistance will promote muscle repair and adaptation. Progressive overload will keep the evolution cycle moving forwards.
C. Raise your NEAT.

Law 3: Satiety and calorie density

Eating foods that make you feel full and satisfied will make controlling your overall caloric intake much easier.

There are many ideas and concepts beyond these laws that you will learn both in this book and on your journey. I call these 5%ers – small details that matter.

Implementing the fundamental laws of change alongside the secondary laws of change will be the key to unlocking your lifelong journey of health.

Yet the science is only half the battle. In order for the science to work, we need to make sure we do it.

This is why we need *The Art of Change*, and that is where we are going next.

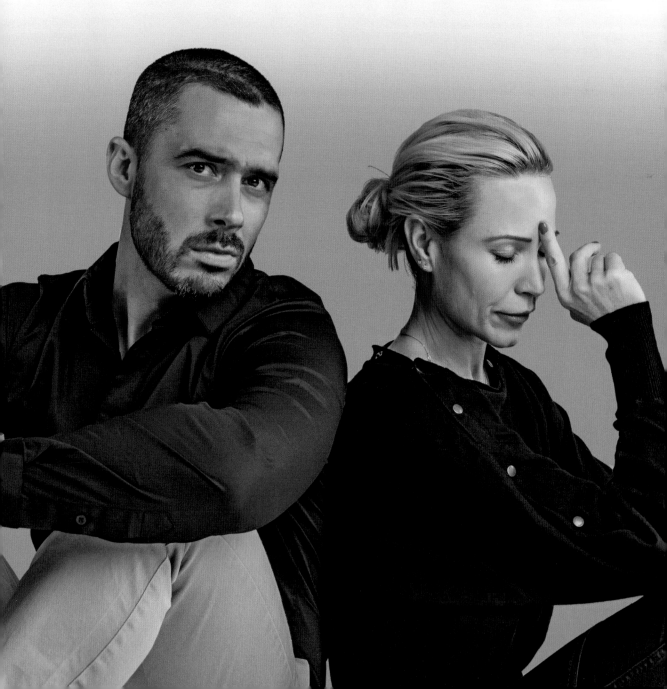

THE ART of CHANGE

INTRODUCTION TO THE ART OF CHANGE

The science of weight loss is simple.

- Understand the basics
- Create a plan based on your goals
- Track your progress and make changes accordingly

However, any coach who claims science has all of the answers to weight management hasn't coached very many people.

As soon as science clashes heads with real people in a normal living environment, the best laid theories of science are put to the ultimate test.

Our infinite complexity and capacity to complicate things is one of the greatest gifts of humanity, it is what makes us interesting, unique and dynamic, but it is also what helps us turn something that is incredibly simple like weight management, into an insurmountable challenge.

Having coached hundreds of people personally, and thousands more remotely, I learned to 'manage' the space between the binary facts of science and those who would to use it to make a change.

I call this space *The Art of Change*. The place where the science meets the reality.

Take the messages in *The Art of Change* as seriously as you do the messages within *The Science of Physical Transformation*.

This is where we marry the simplicity of scientific fact with the complexity of the mind.

Oversimplifying this challenge would be dangerous, but overcomplicating it would be even more dangerous still.

While we should never overcomplicate the process of health and weight management, we shouldn't underestimate the challenges it will present either. Nobody has ever achieved their goals without overcoming many hurdles on the way.

By showing respect to our 'complicated' self, rather than discarding the internal and seemingly unreasonable conflict that can exist within us, we open the door to our ultimate success.

The Art of Change does not pretend to provide therapy or 'fix' the mind, it only intends to help you engage in healthy behaviours.

Of the many thousands of people I have coached from various walks of life – infinitely different personalities, vocations, life experiences and perspectives – each one who succeeded in perpetuity used the philosophies and habits within these pages.

Notice I said 'philosophies and habits'. Not traits.

People who succeed are not 'motivated' and people who fail are not 'lazy' or lacking in 'willpower'.

Motivation, willpower and laziness are all perceived 'traits' and traits are not relevant to your success.

I would not be so bold to claim any of the concepts within these chapters as my own; they are the observations I have made of those who succeeded; observations that have accumulated throughout my career.

As the lessons learned from these observations mounted, I passed this learned insight on to others facing the same challenges and chasing the same goals.

Through this process of cumulative learning I've been able to ensure the next person in line has a far greater chance of succeeding than the one before, until finally, I can be confident that the next person has all of the information they need to succeed.

You are the next person in line.

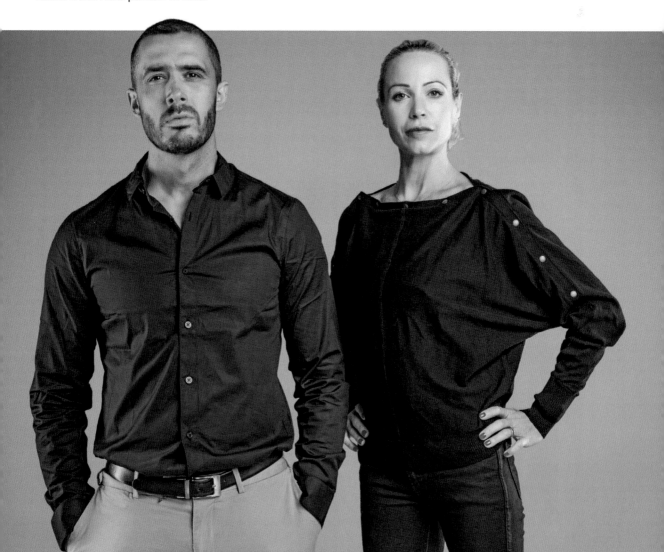

THE IMPORTANCE OF HABITS

If you want to become healthy, habits are everything, yet healthy habits will never become the automatic processes you may expect and even hope them to be.

While some habits are automatic, like picking our noses or swearing in unsuitable situations, many other habits are not.

Healthy habits are manual processes that we prioritize because either:

- A.   The consequences of them matter to us
- B.   They bring us pleasure

Brushing your teeth every morning falls into A.

Unless you have a tooth brush fetish, when you brush your teeth you probably don't take great pleasure from it. If you did not care about whether your teeth fell out, breath smelt or gums receded, you would almost certainly stop brushing your teeth, regardless of how ingrained the habit it was.

A habit that you have held for a lifetime would be deemed superfluous overnight if it no longer held any perceived benefit and the consequences were irrelevant.

On the other hand, if the potato chips you eat every evening while watching TV suddenly tasted like old boots, you would break this habit because it failed to bring you any of the pleasure it once did.

You have a 'habit' of going to work every day, but if your boss announced that you would no longer be paid, you may joyfully break that particular habit there and then.

Habits are central to everything when it comes to health, but healthy habits are not automatic processes. You will not develop an automatic habit because you have done it for one week, four weeks or even 10 years.

You will proceed with a habit because:

- A.   The consequences of them matter to you
- B.   They bring you pleasure

If you can develop a habit that does both, you are winning the habit battle.

Since we can assume you care about the consequences of healthy eating and exercise as you are reading this book:

- •   If you can enjoy exercise, moving your body and working out that gives you a B and an A.
- •   If you enjoy eating healthy foods and the energy they bring you, that gives you a B and an A.

Our first goal is finding ways for you to enjoy exercise and healthy eating. This paradigm shift away from health as 'punishment' and towards 'nourishment' is central to long-term success, but it doesn't end there. This is not the same as enjoying the results.

Many people enjoy the results they achieve but not the way they are achieving them and these habits fall away upon reaching their goals. You need to work rigorously at enjoying the gift of movement and finding new ways to delight your palate with healthy foods.

Non-negotiable

The carefully camouflaged secret behind retaining long-term habits is combining enjoyment with non-negotiable engagement when the pleasure temporarily falls away.

Some days you will not get any pleasure from working out or eating healthily no matter how hard you try.

On these days it is important to remember there is no invisible force that will make your habit occur 'automatically', no matter how long you've done it for.

You retain this habit because the consequences matter to you, but also because you placed it into your hierarchy of non-negotiable manual habits.

You probably don't have a visible non-negotiable manual habits table, but I can guarantee you have them!

TASK

Make a list of habits in your life that you will not negotiate on. These are manual habits that do not get 'managed out' of your priority list.

Then put 'exercise' and 'healthy eating' in there!

Example hierarchy of non-negotiable habits

- Brush and floss my teeth
- Eat more than 70% healthy foods
- Have a bath
- Pay the bills
- Exercise for 30 minutes
- Go to work
- Walk 5,000 steps
- Read to the kids at night
- Walk the dog
- Call mum twice a week
- Have a date night

Harry's Habits 1

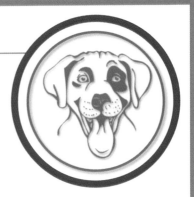

This is Harry.

He **really** wants you to succeed and knows that mindset habits are just as important as exercise and health habits. Every time he sees a habit he likes, he barks, wags his tail, then goes and sits at his computer to type it into this box.

He just found his first habit... about habits... he has a habit of doing that! Down boy!

- **Make healthy habits non-negotiable**

Habit types

If you miss a meal, eat some bad food or snack on some junk one evening, in the scheme of your results, it is almost entirely irrelevant and should be ignored, thrown away and forgotten about.

What changes your body is the habits you keep.

I am less concerned with the ice-cream you ate on a whim at the park, and more concerned with the daily morning latte you have to get going in the morning or the double gin and tonic you drink to relax every evening after work.

Convincing you to avoid the ice-cream you have on a whim every couple of weeks will make almost zero difference to your overall results.

Convincing you to change your latte to a black espresso, or to have a single gin and tonic instead of a double, will significantly alter your results over a period of months.

Don't beat yourself up about making 'mistakes', just don't let them become habits.

Rather than worrying about the few times you 'mess up', think about the daily habits you have that could be replaced with healthier habits without impacting your life in any significant way.

That will make the difference.

Consider your daily habits and how they fit into the following six behaviour types.

Habit types

A.   **Sustainable healthy habit** – a daily occurrence that becomes part of life. This ought to be the main focus of any health plan (daily workout, eating vegetables, drinking water, portion management, walking).

B.   **Consistent unhealthy habit** – a daily occurrence that damages long-term results. Removing these should be the main focus of any health plan (daily junk food, sedentary behaviour, emotional eating).

C.   **Planned unhealthy habit** – a regular habit that is part of your plan. Yes PART OF YOUR PLAN. YOU decide when and how often you eat 'unhealthy' foods, kick back on the couch, have a glass of wine, etc. This is an important part of any long-term health plan.

D.   **Decelerator** – a one-off, undesirable behaviour, the impact of which is overestimated. It will actually have little impact if a one-off. Stopping it becoming a consistent unhealthy habit is the key (missing a workout, giving in to a craving and eating a cake, etc).

E.   **Conscious accelerator** – a planned, healthy behaviour that is understood to not be sustainable, but is implemented in the short-term to accelerate results (double workout, lowering carb intake, removing planned unhealthy habit, etc.).

F.   **Unconscious accelerator** – a behaviour that is seen to be positive but is entirely unsustainable (super-low carb diet, unsustainable total abstinence, overtraining).

These are dangerous behaviours that often result in rebound behaviours.

Success

Find a balance between implementing A, removing B and balancing C that is sustainable for you.

Let the occasional D go (without allowing it to become a B), use E sparingly for accelerating results and avoid F if you want your results to last more than a few months.

NO MORE DIETS

A dieting mindset is not a winning mindset. While it may bring about short-term change it often results in rebound behaviour and unsustainable change.

At the head of your mindset and approach to your healthy life should be exactly that; an approach to a healthy life. It shouldn't be seen as a short-term approach to change, but a lifestyle choice that is important to you.

Case study – There is no wagon

Amanda had been dieting for most of her adult life. When she was dieting, she considered herself to be 'on the wagon' and when she was not dieting, she considered herself to be 'off the wagon'. Her life had proceeded like this for most of her 49 years. I'd been training Amanda for six months when she delightfully announced to me one day:

"I've been on the wagon for six months. This is the longest I've ever stayed on the wagon for. I've been good for that entire time. Soon I'll reach my goals and I can't wait."

"Wait for what?" I asked.

Amanda paused, thought about my question and suddenly looked unsure.

"Actually, I'm a little scared about what happens when I reach my goals. I'm scared about getting off the wagon."

I questioned further. "What is it you're afraid of when you get off the wagon?"

Amanda answered. "There is temptation everywhere. I don't know what I'm going to do when I'm allowed to eat whatever I want again and don't have exercise to distract me every day."

At this point I became concerned. "Amanda, get off that wagon right now. There is no wagon."

"I can't get off the wagon, Daniel. I'm not ready." Hidden in her wagon, she wasn't exposed to temptation. In her mind, she was in a healthy wagon on a fast track journey to Health City. The problem was there was no such place as Health City.

Health is not a journey with a destination, it is a permanent lifestyle choice. Believing in health as a destination is a philosophy ingrained in dieting culture. Once Amanda realized there was no wagon, she was able to focus on creating a long-term balanced lifestyle of health.

Every decision you make, every food you eat, both healthy and unhealthy, every workout you do, every step you take and every rest must be infused with the spirit of permanence.

Transform for Life is not a diet, it is a focus on a permanent healthy lifestyle.

Harry's Habits 2

Harry's happy.

He just found another mindset habit that will help you achieve your goals. He also found a sock that made him happier still...he's easy to please.

- Make healthy habits non-negotiable
- **Focus on a permanent lifestyle change**

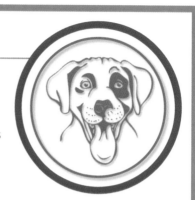

Change your philosophy

Old philosophy: I am on a diet to lose weight.
A diet to lose weight ends in weight loss and then a return to old behaviours once you've achieved your goals.

New philosophy: I am living a healthy lifestyle.
A healthy lifestyle is permanent and continuous.

Old philosophy: I can have that ice cream when I've lost 10lb.
Restriction and avoidance is a behaviour that results in 'yo-yo' behaviours.

New philosophy: I can eat everything I enjoy, provided it is not in excess.
It may be easier to engage in complete avoidance in the early stages of making a change, but to live a permanent healthy life you will need to learn to enjoy foods that are important to you in moderation.

Old philosophy: I am being good.
Being 'good', assumes you can also be 'bad'. This rise and fall is another reason so many fail.

New philosophy: I am living a healthy lifestyle.
You are building a healthy lifestyle. The further you move towards sustainability, the easier your adaptation to permanence.

Old philosophy: I should exercise and eat healthily.
You shouldn't do anything. Every decision in life comes with a consequence and an outcome; It is your choice if health and weight management are important to you.

New philosophy: I choose to nourish my body.
Nourish your body with healthy foods that enrich your life and support your dreams and ambitions. Gift your body with movement that it loves, appreciates and pays you back tenfold for.

FALSE BELIEFS

False beliefs are strange things. We hold on to information that is not true because we have created a story that we tell ourselves. Sometimes we've told ourselves the story for so long we are no longer able to see past it.

There are vast books written on this complex subject, yet at the core of letting go of false beliefs is questioning them and recognizing them not to be true.

Phrases like '*I always give up*' or '*I lose motivation*' are examples of strong and damaging false beliefs that need correcting in various ways.

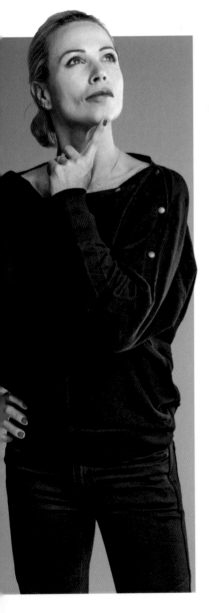

Layla, 64, on 'always giving up'

Perhaps I gave up on something early in my childhood, I can't even remember now, but at some point I decided I gave up on things and this became my story, not just with my health, but with everything.

Every time I gave up, it probably strengthened my belief in this story.

When I met Daniel and he heard me use this language, he questioned me immediately.

He explained that I was writing my own future before it had begun, using the past as a template, rather than using the wealth of information and experiences I learned in the past to change the outcome.

Now, I do not 'always give up'.

I've decided 'I never give up'. I like that story better. This story is as true as I choose to make it. For the last 17 months at least, it has been true.

Beliefs versus truths

Belief: I don't have enough time.

Truth: We all have the exact same amount of time available to us, it's how we choose to spend it. You have enough time. Health needs to be a priority.

Belief: I can't lose weight because I have a slow metabolism.

Truth: Your metabolism may be slower than others, making weight loss slightly more challenging, but the amount of exercise you do, the amount of food you eat and your daily activity levels all play a far greater role in your weight than your baseline metabolic rate.

Belief: I want to succeed but I can't give up the foods I love.

Truth: Who said you have to give up the foods you love? Just eat them a little less often.

Belief: I have a bad ankle/hand/shoulder. I'll start when I get better.

Truth: You could start today. There are very few injuries that stop you doing some form of exercise and none that stop you eating a healthy diet.

Belief: I don't have any discipline.

Truth: Yes you do. Discipline is a choice. You can make that choice the same as anybody else.

Belief: I have to take care of others before myself.

Truth: When we look after ourselves we are better people for those we care about. Every single person who works out and eats healthily tells me it has a positive impact on the relationships that matter to them.

Belief: I always give up so I will only give up again.

Truth: If you always allow your past to shape your future, your future is already written. You are a different person today than you were yesterday. Provided you don't allow the past to shape your future, anything is possible.

Belief: As soon as I eat chocolate/cake/pizza I can't stop.

Truth: You will have moments when you eat pizza, cake and chocolate. You have a choice, you can make a good one. There is no invisible force, just you and your capacity for choice.

Harry's Habits 3

Harry's happy.

He just found another mindset habit that will help you achieve your goals. He also found a roll of toilet paper...Harry loves toilet paper.

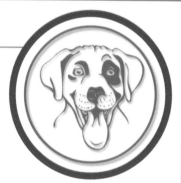

- Make healthy habits non-negotiable
- Focus on a permanent lifestyle change
- **Question false beliefs**

TASK

The line in the sand.

Draw an imaginary line on the floor.

Stand by this line and imagine that every single moment in your life happened on one side of this line.

This side represents your past.

Your memories, your experiences, your successes and your failures.

The other side of the line belongs to your future, as yet unwritten, and endlessly stretching out in undetermined directions and with infinite possibilities.

Now stand on the line.

The line is now. The present moment. The only reality we can ever know. On this line we shape our lives. It is just as impossible to take strides in our future as it is to exist again in our past.

As you stand on this line, you stand between two distinct worlds: the world of the past and the world of the future.

Now you have a choice to make.

1. You can walk over the line facing the past, walking BACKWARDS into your own future.

Instead of looking at a world of opportunity, possibility and change, every moment you create is based on previous experience. Every step crafted with the help of an endless tapestry of familiarity and certainty.

It has happened before, thus it shall happen again.

You are holding up a mirror for the future to create its reality, using a reflection of the past as a guide.

When you face the past as you move to the future, your future is already written and your beliefs will be true.

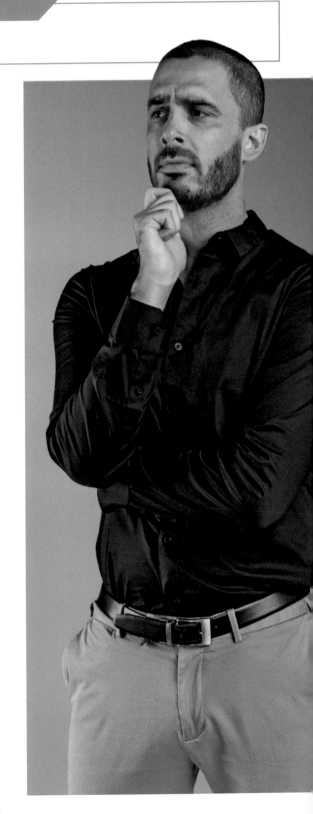

"I have no self control," you tell yourself as you try to avoid eating 'junk' food. While trying to change your behaviour, you are simultaneously watching your previous experiences on repeat and showcasing them to your future.

Your future success is being hijacked by what you believe to be true but which is a false belief.

These experiences were in a different environment, with different circumstances and approached by a different person.

If you keep showing re-runs of your own life to your future, it is indeed a certainty that the future will reflect the past. It could be no other way.

2. Turn around.

Every morning, stand on the distinct line that separates the two worlds that define us. What you have done and what you are yet to do.

You can reflect on the past, collecting the memories and experiences that matter and discarding those that don't. Learn from the past as a wealth of experiences, rather than using it as a template for the future. Turn around and face the future stretching out in front of you, yet to be written and free of constraints, accompanied by the positive experiences and memories you choose to hold on the journey.

You are governed by choice, not by what has gone before.

Position your canvas, amass your paints, mix new colours, formulate new shapes and sculpt new outcomes, with the infinite possibilities of a small child on their first day of school.

Walk forwards with your eyes on the horizon. There is nothing you can't achieve and nothing that can't be done.

HEALTH AND HAPPINESS

Vicky, 32, A letter to herself.

You've always told yourself you have a choice. You can be happy, or you can be healthy.

"I'll never be healthy, I love food too much". How many times have you said that, Vicky?

But it's a lie isn't it?

Because you do not love the food that made you gain weight, you were addicted to it. Living a life where you believed it made you happy. You have never loved food as much as you do now. Healthy, fresh, delicious food.

Once the fog of dependence clears, healthy food is left, and ironically that's helping to make you healthy.

Remember this. Because things are good at the moment, you are focused. You're focused on cooking, being in control, exercising. Feeling better, working towards a positive future.

Remember that this is now your path for life.

Remember these things, when the diversion happens, to get you back on your path at the nearest entrance.

I write this letter to you because I don't want you to buy the lie that you are 'happier' when you're eating excesses of foods that make you gain weight. You aren't.

You are happier right now, eating a balanced, healthy diet and exercising.

While we can never say with absolute confidence that being healthy will make us happy (if perpetual happiness is even possible), we can say with absolute confidence that eating large amounts of 'unhealthy' foods will not and does not bring long-term contentment.

Most people take a great deal of pleasure from food. They love the taste, the social aspect and the joy that food can bring.

People who take control of their diet and health love food even more; they love healthy food and they love unhealthy food. All the food they eat is consumed guilt free. If you love food, healthy eating will make you love it even more!

Being healthy is a fundamental human need. Eating what we want, when we want goes against this fundamental need, bringing feelings of guilt and diminishing the pleasure.

You can love food, enjoy food, experience food and love life even more when you are healthy.

I have personally coached over 300 people to change and have been involved in the healthy transformation of many thousands, and I am yet to meet a single person who was happier when they were not engaging in healthy behaviours.

Exercise and healthy eating does an awful lot more than it advertises!

Being healthy will usually:

- Bring confidence
- Give you more energy
- Improve your physical appearance
- Improve emotional resilience
- Improve self-esteem
- Improve general mood
- Reduce chance of chronic disease
- Improve life span
- Increase mobility
- Increase contentment levels
- Give you a sense of purpose
- Provide a sense of achievement
- Decrease anxiety and reduce depression

I am fairly certain eating 'junk' food on the couch can't do any of these things for you!

The healthy compromise

While health comes with numerous exciting promises, it is not a magic bullet, and like everything in life worth having, sacrifices must be made.

Making time for health is a choice that permeates almost every aspect of your life in a positive way, but also in ways that may need compromises with other things that matter to you.

Many of our members consider this compromise to be the most important aspect of their ultimate success.

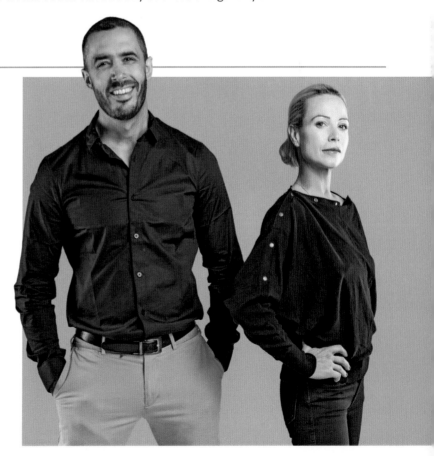

COMPARISON

Individuality

Imagine, if you will, living in a world, where every one of us is identical.

In this sanitized version of humanity, each and every person would exactly match the 'perfect' ideal.

In this world, the word 'individual' has not been used for thousands of years. Redundant. Superfluous. Banished to history.

Voices freed of all chance or need to discover new harmonies.

No body, no face and no opinion could differ, because any slight deviation would contradict the fabric of this society. Intrinsically, perfection has only one version.

The perfect version.

Would this theoretical civilization have reached the pinnacle of mankind?

Perfection.

All citizens looking, thinking and functioning in exactly the same way.

The perfect way.

GET ME OUT OF THERE! NOW!

Free of this homogeneous prison, remember that in our world, your body, your face and your mind is different to mine and celebrate.

We spend so much time comparing and judging that we forget that the differences in ourselves that we berate are actually the greatest gifts we own.

Because different is incalculably better than perfection.

To be unique is infinitely preferable to being ideal.

Being diverse is immeasurably more satisfying than being uniform.

You are not perfect and neither am I. The most wondrous trait we share is that we manifest incomparability in every way.

Ask yourself the following question, free from rhetoric, sentiment and cliché:

Is there anything more beautiful in this universe than the beauty of oneness?

Oneness in the sense that we share it all.

Oneness in that we are the only one.

Comparing how many workouts you do, how fit you are, or how tough you find things will offer no benefit to your journey and most likely will damage it.

Some of us may be fitter than others, some of us are younger, some of us are older, some of us can do more press ups, some can do more squats, some are great with cardio, some are great with resistance. It's all irrelevant.

What matters is that you are the best you!

We travel together. We walk the path of fitness together as equals on the same road!

The only comparison you should make is to the you of yesterday.

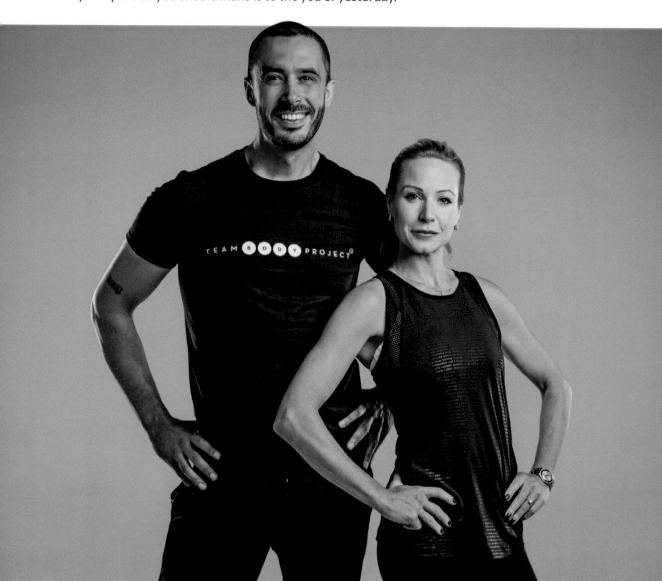

The IMPOSSIBLE comparison

Comparison to others is just about the most pointless, demotivating and false thing you could ever do.

If you compare your fitness to another persons, you are making a comparison of a single aspect of your lives - yet our lives are diverse and impossible to measure against one another.

Another person may have good fitness, but you don't know how they are faring in other aspects of their life.

They may have damaged relationships, unfulfilled travel ambitions, financial difficulties and numerous other factors that are challenging them.

They may have had more opportunities in life than you, or they may have had less opportunities.

They may have had more luck than you, or perhaps they've had less luck. Who knows?

Unless you know every single variable in another persons life and background - any comparison you make is not just damaging and pointless, it is also empirically incorrect:

> A.   The focus is too narrow to be a true comparison
> B.   The hierarchy of factors will be different

They may care more about health, you may care more about politics, charity or even money and possessions. Who are we to judge which factors matter the most?

Therefore, the ONLY person you can ever confidently measure yourself against, is yourself.

Are you fitter than you were yesterday?
Are you kinder than you were last month?
Are you less anxious than you were last week?
Are you a better YOU?

The answer to these questions may not always be positive - progress will oscillate throughout your life and numerous factors will influence it, but at least you are making a fair assessment:

> A.   The comparison is a true one
> B.   You CAN always make tomorrow a little bit better than today

Comparison to others must be thrown out of the equation if we are to make the very best of ourselves.

Harry's Habits 4

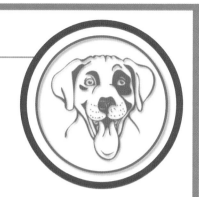

Harry's happy.

He just found another mindset habit that will help you achieve your goals. He also discovered he has a tail so he's been chasing that for a while.

- Make healthy habits non-negotiable
- Focus on a permanent lifestyle change
- Question false beliefs
- **Don't compare yourself to others**

Comparison to self

Starting with a health and workout routine should be a most rejuvenating experience, but it can also be a demotivating one.

Why?

We all have benchmarks and standards by which we hold ourselves and when starting a health regime, the realization of how far from your personal peak you are can do more harm than good.

While some feel the fuels burning bright when the realizations hit, an equal, if not higher number, feel overwhelmed by this newly found cognizance.

In some ways it is easier to accept your differences with others than it is to accept a failure to live up to personal expectations, which, by virtue of being distinctly particular to self, are within reach.

If we can't run as fast as Usain Bolt, dance like Fred Astaire or sing like Aretha Franklin, it's easy to explain this away, but it's far more complex and infinitely less easy to explain why we don't achieve our own personal best.

How do we square something we know to be a circle?

As discussed previously, there is certainly a benefit to holding oneself up against personal expectation. Without it we can not have ambition, aspiration or progress, so how do we come to terms with negative comparisons to our previous self?

We focus on the successes, rather than the outcomes, at least in the short term.

Judgement of self is often better confined to the actions of today than to the circumstances that may or may not have been created by the actions of yesterday, or to the perceptions of where we believe we should be tomorrow.

- Did you workout today?
- Did you eat healthily today?
- Did you drink plenty of water today?

Yes?

You're a winner!

The actions you took today are the actions of a champion! That person is somebody to be proud of and that person will certainly become the best version of themselves.

KINDNESS

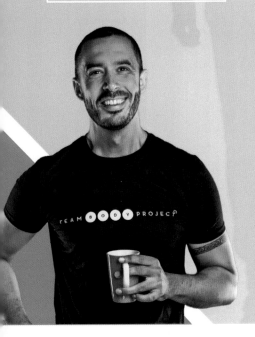

> Life was ROCK BOTTOM, unthinkable thoughts were circulating in my mind faster than I could process them.

I was having my morning coffee in a cafe that I visited almost every day throughout my early twenties.

I had never felt worse than I did on this particular day, yet to look at my expression you probably wouldn't have known it.

Life was rock bottom, unthinkable thoughts were circulating in my mind faster than I could process them. If 'coping' lived in the North Pole, I'd planted my flag at the South.

For the previous few months, I had noticed an elderly lady feeding seeds to the birds in a churchyard opposite where I was sitting.

We'd never spoken nor even acknowledged one another, yet I'd always noticed her, patiently feeding and caring for these birds, and had often wondered what her story might be.

This particular morning, I didn't notice her until she was stood in front of me. Her face was worn and marked by wrinkled skin betraying a lifetime of exposure to bleak weather and hardships untold.

Some things stand out because they don't belong, like a flower in full bloom in the midst of winter. Her face was old and haggard, yet when she looked at me, I was stunned by her eyes, that were clear and youthful.

And then, she whispered four simple words.

'It will be alright.'

That was it.

She turned to feed the birds she fed every morning and I never saw her again.

She spoke only four words to me yet influenced my life more than people who have spoken hundreds of thousands. She chose her words wisely.

She could have said, "Cheer up, it might never happen" or 'You look like you've got the weight of the world on your shoulders."

But she didn't. She said, "It will be alright." And in doing so, planted a seed that would grow into a powerful belief.

Kindness matters. Words matter.

Even a stranger can change a life if they use the right words.

This lady may not know that she had such a profound impact on my life, but then again, maybe she does.

Unkind comments

Making negative comments about another persons body is unkind and profoundly unhelpful OR demonstrates an extraordinary lack of self awareness. If anybody does make comments about your body that are anything but kind, remember this:

1. It says far more about their uneducated attitude towards health than it does about your body.
2. Very few people make positive changes because of negative criticism (although some do - but it VERY seldom sustains)
3. Most people make permanent positive change from a position of learned confidence, support and kindness

Feel confident in your body today; show it the positive attention and kindness it deserves.

Kindness drives positive action!

While many negative comments (often from family and friends) may be dressed as concern, comments such as these frequently cause eating disorders, mental health issues and extreme behaviours. Without these remarks, anorexia, bulimia, body dysmorphia and a whole plethora of body image disorders, conditions, mental health issues and self-esteem issues would not receive the oxygen they need to exist.

Let others know you will never judge them for their appearance and you will positively support their choices. And expect the same of them.

Kindness to self

Don't workout because you hate your body, workout because you love your body.

One of the saddest truths of all is that we reserve our least kind words for ourselves.

Saying cruel and damaging words to ourselves many times a day will negatively impact our goals, our mindset and our state of mind.

Choose the words you use when speaking to yourself carefully, as if it were somebody you cared about and loved that you were speaking with.

Don't wait until you reach your goals to be kind to yourself, start it now.

Like everything else in this book, the more you do it, the better you will become at it.

Harry's Habits 5

Harry's happy.

He just found another mindset habit that will help you achieve your goals. He also heard the word "walk" from 200 yards out of earshot.

- Make healthy habits non-negotiable
- Focus on a permanent lifestyle change
- Question false beliefs
- Don't compare yourself to others
- **Be kind to yourself**

Kindness to self

1. Whenever you hear or create a negative thought about yourself, try not to dwell on it.

2. Create a new thought about yourself that focuses on a positive aspect of your personality or body.

3. Treat this process the same as any other habit.

4. The conscious effort of being kind to yourself will, over time, become a larger part of your subconscious.

5. However, being kind to yourself needs work and application every day, just like exercise and nutrition.

Progress is better than change

When you reach your goal weight you will be the same person as you are now. Lighter, fitter and healthier, but the same person.

While the process of transforming your body will be one that improves every element of your life, it will not change who you are.

Be kind to yourself as you move forwards and make progress towards your goals.

The progress you see in your habits, your mindset and the way you approach your health is worth celebrating and congratulating daily. This progress is more important than ultimate change, because it keeps on coming and can be measured regularly.

- Every time you make a positive decision is progress
- Every time you workout is progress
- Every time you eat a healthy meal is progress
- Every time you don't dwell on a negative thought is progress
- Every time you are kind to yourself is progress
- Every time you don't give in to emotional eating is progress

Celebrate every moment of progress on your journey. (*The non-scale victory* chapter coming up will help you do this.)

The human mind is like Teflon for positive information, slipping away without ever really being felt or acknowledged, and like Velcro for negative information, sticking to the sides until forcefully pulled off. This is the human condition. It is the same experience for all of us. If we are to give the same or more acknowledgement to our victories as our failures, we must do it consciously.

The process of acknowledging the positive and removing the negative must be practised, worked on and developed into a habit.

Harry's Habits 6

Harry's happy.

He just found another mindset habit that will help you achieve your goals. He also dug up a bone whilst burying one of his owner's slippers.

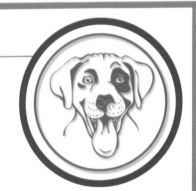

- Make healthy habits non-negotiable
- Focus on a permanent lifestyle change
- Question false beliefs
- Don't compare yourself to others
- Be kind to yourself
- **Celebrate every victory**

CORE MINDSET HABITS

The mindset fundamentals in the previous chapters have varying levels of relevance and resonance to those who read them.

The core mindset habits are held by nearly everybody who succeeds at lifetime health.

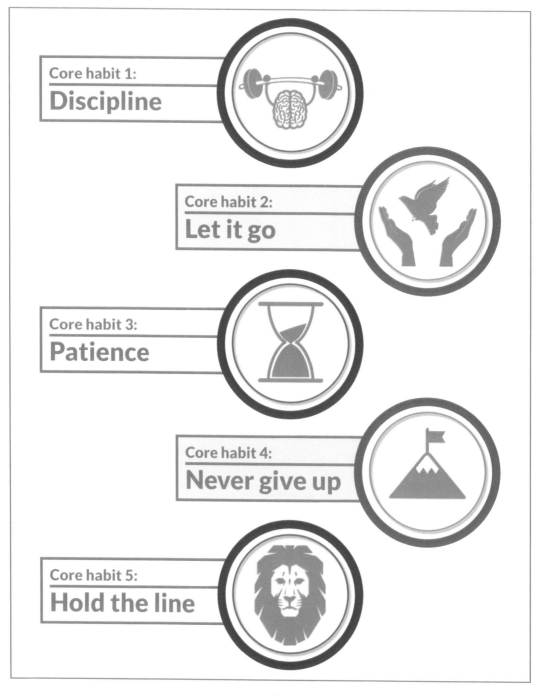

Core habit 1:
Discipline

Core habit 2:
Let it go

Core habit 3:
Patience

Core habit 4:
Never give up

Core habit 5:
Hold the line

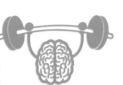

DISCIPLINE VERSUS MOTIVATION - CORE HABIT 1

When you start the *Transform for Life* plan, with fresh goals and excitement at what lies ahead, you may feel a tingle in your stomach, a spring in your step and hope in your heart.

That feeling is called motivation. You feel like you could take on the world.

This feeling, motivation, is actually a dangerous opponent in your journey to a lifetime of health and the greatest foe in creating new habits and breaking old ones because if you are not careful, you will learn to give motivation the glory when you succeed and blame its absence when you do not.

When you make a mistake during your health plan and motivation abandons you (motivation always abandons you when you make a mistake) you will feel like a failure, like you let motivation down.

This may cause you to turn a small irrelevant mistake into a series of mistakes.

I have seen motivation ruin more health plans than any other thing during all my years as a coach.

Bust the motivation myth

Today, I am going to be the kid in the playground who told you Santa Claus does not exist. I am going to be the parent you caught putting a coin underneath your pillow instead of the tooth fairy.

You will NEVER feel motivated every day.

The motivation you may feel now, you will lose. It will return and then fade again because that is what motivation does. It hangs around for a while to give you a healthy boost and then it disappears into the sunset, taking your goals with it!

Perpetual motivation is a myth and anybody vending it is selling a product no more useful than snake oil.

It has let down millions of people around the world who believe in its mystical powers and give up when it abandons them, or worse still, blame themselves.

Motivation will abandon you, so dump it before it dumps you!

Factor	Root determinant	Reliability
Motivation	Feeling	Poor
Discipline	Choice	Absolute

The truth about success

Like it or not, to succeed you are going to have to learn to workout when you don't feel like it and eat healthily when the going gets tough.

Exercise

- Everybody can workout when they're motivated. Those who succeed workout when they're NOT motivated.

Nutrition

- Everybody can eat healthy when the going is good. Those who succeed eat healthy when the going gets tough.

I want the following truth-bomb to hit you hard in the face. The harder it hits you, the better.

You WILL NOT ACHIEVE YOUR GOALS if you rely on MOTIVATION.

I'd rather say it now so we can prepare for that hurdle in advance. If you rely on the motivation you are feeling now to succeed in achieving your goals then you won't achieve your goals.

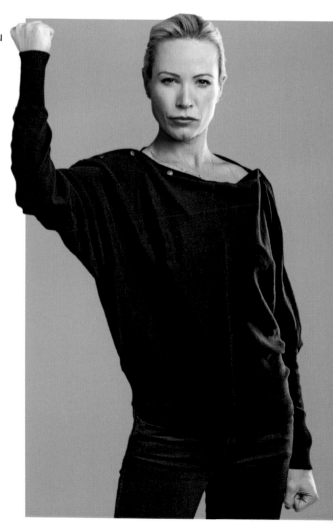

Your success will have nothing to do with motivation and everything to do with discipline.

Discipline is not a thing we have or do not have. It is not a gift or a trait or a special ability. It is the capacity to follow a plan.

With *Transform for Life* we give you a plan.

Discipline is not special or unique or mystical. It is the choice to do something we decide we are going to do.

You are as disciplined as me and I am as disciplined as you.

Discipline is a choice.
Motivation is a feeling.

My favourite four words in the English language again, and words that changed my own life once I learned them:

Discipline is a choice.

Discipline works. Discipline isn't sexy, it's routine.

It's Dickensian and it's boring but it works and never lets you down.

You will have bad days, you will make mistakes, you will miss workouts, you will lose motivation and, yes, you will lose discipline.

The difference between motivation and discipline is choice. We must wait for motivation to come and find us, while discipline waits for us to come and find it.

Changing your body and changing your habits is going to be hard.

There are going to be days when you don't enjoy it, you don't feel like it and want to give up.

We want to believe in motivation because we know how powerful it would be. If only we could feel motivated every day, but we can't, so we have to rely on something that will work.

The motivation turnover

Most people consider motivation to be a 'push' to action.
Those who succeed know that action is a 'pull' to motivation.

Case study – Mary, 43

I had always thought I lacked motivation and those who succeeded were simply more motivated to do it than I was.

About six weeks into my 'latest' health plan, I turned up to a boxing class with Daniel and explained I'd lost all motivation. It always happened to me after a few weeks and I was expecting him to be disappointed and try and cheer me up.

In fact he didn't even try and motivate or cheer me up even a little bit, instead he just pleaded with me to take part in the boxing class anyway. In truth, I was a bit disappointed he had.

I reluctantly did the class. Normally I would have just gone home.

At the end of the class, I was buzzing and felt really great. Daniel approached me smiling.

"You've just learned the secret of motivation, haven't you?" he said.

I felt good, but didn't quite know what he was getting at.

"Discipline," he said with a grin.

At that moment it clicked for me.

Motivation wasn't something that pushed me to do something.
Doing something pulled me into feeling motivated again!

The workouts you do when 'don't feel like it' and when motivation evades you are the most important workouts you do.

The discipline shown to workout when we are demotivated accelerates motivation turnover. In other words, it brings motivation back faster.

We shouldn't reject the concept of motivation altogether because, when there, it's a nice bonus.

We should just give it no credit or place within our health plan.

Just press play

This is the central philosophy at Team Body Project.

- What you 'feel' like doing is driven by motivation
- What you 'choose' to do is driven by discipline

One works all the time and one works some of the time.

You can tell which one a person hangs their hat on by one simple factor; whether they succeed in achieving their health goals.

For all the mindset techniques, philosophies and habits we can apply, nothing beats *Just Press Play* for simple effectiveness.

The motivational guru

Many years ago I attended a seminar held by a famous motivational guru.

Waiting for him to appear, hundreds of eager attendees sat in an anticipation that could only be quenched by his appearance on stage. The crowd erupted as he stepped into view, his presence as electrifying as it was enthralling.

Larger than life, he proceeded to inspire us with expertly constructed psychobabble.

His mission? To ignite the vast contingent of hopefuls in attendance into realizing how brilliant life was.

I'm normally a deeply analytical man but felt stupid not to join in with such hysteria playing out around me, and besides, I really didn't want to miss out on the promised waves of success.

"Life should be wonderful every moment of every day," he declared.

"YES, IT SHOULD," we responded.

"Every day, ANYTHING is possible," he proclaimed.

"YES, IT IS," we chanted.

"If you dream big enough you can achieve your wildest dreams," he trumpeted at great volume across the room as appropriate, uplifting music played in the background.

"YES, WE CAN," we sang out together.

Surrounded by his energy, and the energy of those around us, we had been roused into a frenzied state of collective delusions of grandeur. The impressively intelligent man to my left declared he WOULD be the next Steve Jobs – I believed him.

"You'll not be the next Steve Jobs," I said, with a twinkle in my eye. "You're much better than that."

He laughed, but his laugh was ironic, his achievements in computing would make the Apple Mac look like a winning prize in a primary school technology competition.

To my left, an outlandishly creative fashion designer exuded confidence as she spoke about creating a brand that would leave Armani quivering in her wake.

And me? I would inspire the whole world to get moving. Bad health would be a thing of the past!

"You're the best!" they both said. I nodded. They were right. I WAS the best.

I beat my chest like a silverback gorilla in mating season and let out an almighty war cry. They were clearly impressed with this newly demonstrated form of expressing oneself and joined in enthusiastically.

We were MOTIVATED.

"Let's meet in six months," I suggested. "Come and visit me at my beach villa in the Maldives."

We laughed, but we knew it was true.

Six months later, I felt embarrassed to invite two such (surely) successful people to a tiny bedsit in a downmarket London district so suggested we meet in a coffee shop in a smart upmarket district.

I scraped together a few coins by scouring the back of my sofa and turning my old jeans upside down. When I arrived, I was a more than a little surprised by the low energy levels they were both displaying.

Mr. Future Apple was in a period of restructuring / aligning his vision.

Mrs. Future Armani was in the process of creating a new line of clothing that she wasn't quite ready for the world to see.
Me? I'd been very busy watching re-runs of The Fresh Prince of Bel-air and eating biscuits in my pyjamas, but told them I was in a period of transition.

We all nodded enthusiastically at our collective attempts to feign success.

Finally, it was Mr. Future Apple who said it.

"I don't know about you guys, but I haven't actually felt that great every day. I was so motivated during the seminar but as soon as I left, 'it' left."

It's a funny thing. The brain thinks it knows what it is true until it hears genuine authenticity. When the real truth plays its unquestionable tune, you just know and suddenly the mistruths that went before them hit the dud notes they always had, except now, you are no longer tone deaf.

Mr. Future Apple was the first person to speak the truth that day.

"Most days I struggle to get going. I REALLY want to be full of energy and motivation like the guy at the seminar, but some days little problems get in the way and I struggle to get going. Other days I feel demotivated and I simply don't know why."

What followed that day was an outpouring of our struggles, of our difficulties, of the barriers that kept being put in our way, that some days it was the most we could do to put one foot in front of the other.

It was at that moment I said something that would change the direction of my life forever.

"What if motivation is just a myth? I do what I love and what I am passionate about. That's meant to be the 'secret', but I STILL don't feel motivated every day. What if the real secret is to try your best when you don't feel motivated?"

That day I learned that other people struggled just as much as me and that there was nothing wrong with my mind or my motivation levels.

I was hindered by a lack of action caused by a falsely perpetuated belief that I should be filled with the joys of spring every day.

And here's another really important lesson: When the chips are down, when life keeps handing you bad cards, it's a little easier to be kind to yourself when you don't live up to your often unrealistic expectations.

What is really difficult to bend your head around is losing motivation and inspiration for no reason. That's the brain twister many of us wrestle with.

When you should be motivated and there is no reason not to be! You start beating yourself up and thinking there is something wrong with you, when of course this is perfectly natural too.

It is normal to feel demotivated for no reason!

On these days, no matter how bad we feel, let us beat our hands on our chest like almighty silverback gorillas in the midst of the mating season and declare: "I'm going to do it anyway."

Discipline does not mean perfect.

The choice to be healthy will confront you every day for the rest of your life.

Believing in discipline does not mean you will make the right choice every day. That's not what discipline is, because life isn't that simple.

We all mess up, make mistakes and go off-track.

Discipline is a philosophy you can return to immediately without guilt, whenever you go off-track. It won't abandon you because you made a mistake.

On the other hand, motivation is a philosophy that punishes you for mistakes by withdrawing its services until it forgives you and comes back.

Whatever your approach in the past, you can take the choice to be disciplined now.

There is nothing more powerful and no feeling more important than the feeling of success that hits you when you 'do it anyway'.

'Active' versus 'contained' discipline

Ever wondered why you are so good at working out every day, but struggle to follow a good diet alongside it?

Active discipline is the discipline to do something.

A person who works out every day demonstrates excellent active discipline.

They show the discipline to do something in the short-term that may not provide instant gratification but does provide longer term benefits.

A person who avoids eating sugar, large portions, drinking alcohol or smoking is showing contained discipline. They are using discipline to not do something.

In my experience, a person who shows excellent active discipline does not necessarily show excellent contained discipline.

The reason many people struggle with achieving the healthy body and results they desire is that success at health requires both types of discipline to be in force, leaving frustration for the regular exerciser who deserves more for their efforts.

Therefore, regular exercisers who show excellent active discipline need to use their capacity for action to drive contained discipline.

How?

People who show strong active discipline are shown to get a surge in feel-good hormones from taking action, which is possibly why they are so successful at taking action.

However, no feel good hormones are released during contained discipline. In fact, when you show contained discipline you are often depriving yourself of (temporary) feel good hormones.

Therefore you need to use active discipline in moments when contained discipline is called for.

As an example; when you are faced with a sugar craving, take the action of drinking a glass of water and maybe even doing 10 'on the spot' squats.

This will both release a few feel good hormones and provide your mind with a reward for taking action. It also takes contained discipline out of the abstract and into the tangible.

In other words, use your capacity for action to become stronger at containing cravings and desires.

LET IT GO – CORE HABIT 2

Under normal circumstances, I don't like ruining surprises.

One Christmas, I went hunting for the presents that my parents had hidden.

Upon finding them, I experienced a fleeting moment of joy as I discovered what delights were awaiting me, followed by a feeling of abject disappointment that I'd ruined the surprise.

There was, however, one distinct advantage to knowing what was waiting for me under the Christmas tree. I knew exactly how I was going to react.

While my brother's face struggled to hold back the disappointment when opening his unwanted and soon discarded Christmas socks, I'd been preparing for this exact moment for weeks.

"Wow Nanna, I've been waiting for a new pair of socks just like these," I said smugly, as my brother looked on in disbelief.

Sometimes, being ready for a surprise has its advantages.

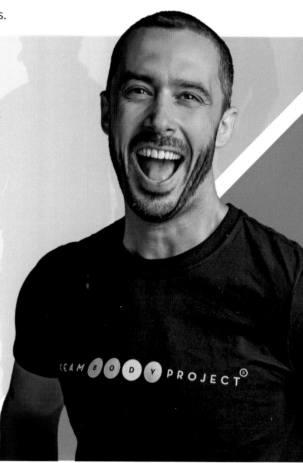

Surprise

On balance, I've decided there are some surprises you are better off hearing now so you're prepared for them.

Surprise 1: You WILL miss a workout.

Surprise 2: You WILL have an unplanned blowout.

You could be the exception to this rule, but most likely you won't be. Nearly everybody makes a mistake and goes off piste on their health plan. Let's have a look at how much it matters.

Factor	Person 1	Total +/-	Person 2	Total +/-
BMR	2,000 kcal x 7 days	14,000 kcal	2,000 kcal x 7 days	14,000 kcal
Calorie intake	1,500 kcal x 7 days	-10,500 kcal	1,500 kcal x 7 days	-10,500 kcal
Food 'mistakes'	Bowl of ice cream	-500 kcal	None	0 kcal
Total calorie deficit		3,000 kcal		3,500 kcal
Exercise	300 kcal x6 workouts	2,100 kcal	300 kcal x6 workouts	2,100 kcal
NEAT	250 kcal x 7 days	1,750 kcal	250 kcal x7 days	1,750 kcal
Missed workouts	250 kcal x2 workouts	-500 kcal	None	0 kcal
Total calorie burn		3,350 kcal		3,850 kcal
Total deficit + burn		6,350 kcal		7,350 kcal
Weight lost*		1.8 lb		2.1 lb

* based on 3,500 kcal being equivalent to 1 lb of weight loss

Person 1 lost just 0.3 lb less than Person 2 despite:

- Missing two workouts
- Eating a large bowl of ice cream

Person 1 could easily think they 'messed up' this week, while person 2 could be very happy with themselves.

In truth, the results they experienced were almost identical. The physiological difference is entirely negligible. However the psychological consequences could be catastrophic.

Person 1 can often start to label themselves as:

- Lazy
- Lacking will power
- Having no self-control
- Having no discipline

This attitude could prompt these insignificant events to turn from insignificant events into habits. That will matter.

Eating a bowl of ice cream that you hadn't planned for, missing a workout, bingeing on biscuits or anything else that wasn't part of your plan makes no difference to your overall results whatsoever.

So just *let it go*.

The difference between success and failure will not come down to whether or not you go 'off-piste', because you will.

It will come down to how you respond to it. If you label yourself with falsehoods and tell yourself you can't do it, you will prove yourself right.

If you accept that you are human, fallible and not a robot, you can brush yourself off and carry on, as you were.

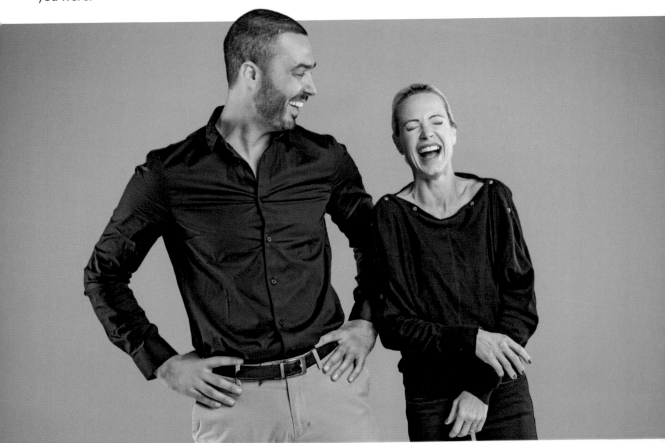

Sunset

In London, you are surrounded in all directions by high rise buildings that unapologetically obstruct the horizon.

Smog and pollution drape a subtle blanket across the sky.

Sunrises and sunsets are replaced by the honking of horns, whirring engines from planes overhead and the hustle and bustle of the day beginning and ending.

While paying lip service to 'seizing the day' I had never fully appreciated what this meant until I spent a few days watching the sun rise to welcome the new day and the sun set to bid it farewell.

The sunset brings clarity to the importance of NOW. Today is the only day like it, no other day like today will ever exist.

The sunset brings with it a chance to reflect on the days failures, successes, opportunities seized and opportunities missed. It is a chance to let it all go with
a smile and look forwards to a new dawn.

'Seize the day' is what we normally take from this… but this is not what I learned.

In distinctly separating each day we are given the chance to let go of mistakes, things we regret and things we didn't get right.

As the sun goes down, we have an opportunity to 'seize closure' on the day that has passed.

If we allow our past to dictate our future, our future is already written.

So while 'seize the day' is popularized in modern culture, I actually believe that 'seizing closure' on the day that has gone before could be THE take away from the circadian cycle that sets natural rhythm to our lives.

By letting go of the past, we free ourselves to seize opportunities that make the difference we want in the new dawn.

PATIENCE – CORE HABIT 3

Patience and peas

At 18 years old, with no discernible skills, meaningful accomplishments or qualifications, I was pretty much unemployable. So when, one summer, I was offered a night job in a pea factory I jumped at the opportunity.

At the start of my first shift the manager of the pea factory enthusiastically led me through his domain, explaining the minutiae of the pea's journey from 'farm to shopping basket' through his fine establishment.

As a newly appointed worker I felt it important to ingratiate myself into the life of the pea and therefore listened intently.

"So what's my role in all of this Mr Peabody?" I asked.

"Ahhh," he replied with a twinkle in his eye. "Come with me, young man."

And so off we plodded through this wonderful land of peas. We ascended what felt like a hundred flights of legume-filled floors until we reached the summit of the factory.

Mount Pea, if you like.

"Here is where the magic starts," Mr Peabody declared, opening his arms towards an enormous shiny bucket.

"The pride and joy of the factory."

Indeed it was. A giant canister, packed to the brim with the greenest and cleanest peas this side of the moon.

"So what do you need me for?" I asked.
"We must get the peas from up HERE... to down THERE."

He gestured beneath us towards waves of conveyor belts, lined with hair-netted workers ready to inspect the peas that were soon to cascade upon them.

"Why don't you just tilt the bucket and pour them?" I asked, with a naïve shrug.

He threw me a knowing look before reaching behind the giant bucket of peas.

"Because the peas must be frozen, so they stay fresh for the customers, young man. When you tilt, they go nowhere, until you break them up with THIS."

It was in this opportune moment, that he handed me a gargantuan silver fork in a short ceremonial gesture that felt like a miniature coronation.

Was he crowning me King of the Peas? But instead of presenting a crown, he was bestowing upon me a giant fork.

I took the gigantic fork into my hands, gazing at it with wonder. I then turned my eyes on the workers below, full of anticipation on the conveyor belts, waiting for the fork to strike its maiden blow and commence proceedings.

Entrusted upon me, on my first day at work, was this, the most important job in the factory. I was the master of the pea universe and nothing would happen until I hefted my almighty fork.

Now, although I was honoured to be given such a role, just five minutes into my first shift I was also cautious, as heavy is the crown.

Even though young, I knew this much.

"He's spotted something in me," I thought to myself. "He's seen something special. I won't let him down, I will be the most honourable bearer of the fork at the summit of Mount Pea there has ever been!"

I turned to Mr Peabody, wiped a tear from my eye and raised my hand to my forehead in full military salute. He saluted me back. We looked in each other's eyes and the gaze was held.

Not a blink was given.

Brave, honourable men can see the resilience in each other's souls when they stare long and deep enough. I imagine it was at this moment that Mr Peabody knew. Although he'd taken an almighty risk on such an unproven candidate, he'd made the right decision.

I gave him the nod.

"Let's get this show on the road..."

And at exactly 10pm on 8th August the pea bucket was tilted, I hefted my almighty fork, striking an unyielding strike into the surface layer and the four tines of the ceremonial weapon sent the perilous peas down towards their dinner destiny.

The factory was back in business with a new master at the helm...

45 minutes later, at exactly 10.45pm, I realized I'd been had.

I was no King.

This was the hardest, most relentless job in the factory. I was the latest in a long line of pea paupers that seldom lasted a night. I had another seven hours of frozen pea crushing to go and my shoulders and back were already numb with pain.

It was the longest night of my life. I didn't take my eyes off the clock all night. Every back-breaking, soul-destroying minute observed as it ticked slowly by.

Yet, the funny thing is, 20-odd years later, I can remember this first ever shift as if it was yesterday.

The strange thing with time is that moments can feel like you are trudging through mud, but years will fly by in a heartbeat.

So why am I regaling this oddly abstract account of an experience from two decades ago, and what on Earth has it got to do with your health?

The number one reason for people giving up on a health plan is impatience with results. I watched the clock every minute of every hour during those fork-hefting night shifts, just as many people watch the scales, the tape measure, the results, every single day of an exercise routine.

Sometimes it feels like it's taking forever. So people QUIT what they were doing so well because it just seems to take so long... because they're watching the clock.

The ensuing months go by in a heartbeat and then they remember they want a healthy body, so they restart again.

If they had never quit with frustration they would now be further along the road, exactly where they wanted to be.

"The days are long but the years are short." – Gretchen Rubin

Whenever you feel like quitting, whenever you feel like it's taking you a long time to get where you want to be, remember that today will become two months, six months, two years, ten years from now in a heartbeat.

So keep focused on today, stop worrying about the results, and remember that all the time you are 'watching the clock' it will feel like it's taking a long time.

Unlike me with my short-lived pea career, if you're working out you're on the right track!

As soon as you take your eyes off the clock, time will fly by and before you know it, it will be the end of your shift.

The shift always ends, just as results always come to those who persist.

Oh and if a kindly fella with a giant fork ever offers you a job... Smile, politely decline and run away as fast as you can.

Patience. Patience. Patience.

There is no greater asset or better habit to exhibit than demonstrating patience in your health journey.

The science of fat loss is exact and precise but it is not entirely linear:

A.   Some weeks the scales and tape will not budge.
B.   Small, sensible adjustments will need to be made.
C.   When it comes to maintenance, slower results are better

Impatience threatens your results.

You are going to *Transform for Life*. If you are 40 years old, that means you have another 35+ years to experience a healthy weight in a body you love.

Even if it takes you a whole year or more to get there, that's 97% of the rest of your life you get to live in a body you want!

You have three options:

A.   Follow the guidelines patiently and achieve your results in good time.
B.   Try and rush the results and risk losing all progress when you rebound.
C.   Get frustrated, give up and go back to where you started, only to start the process all over again.

The only option that works is option A. **Patience.**

If you continue to follow the guidelines in *Transform for Life* it is a certainty you will achieve the healthy body you want faster than you think.

NEVER GIVE UP – CORE HABIT 4

This is my favourite core habit.

I have three young children, and like all parents I hope they have bright futures and fulfilling lives. If I could teach just one philosophy to each of them, the choice would be easy and the same for all three:

"Never give up."

You need this philosophy every single day of your life. Rejection, failure, disappointment and disasters are encountered more commonly than success and acceptance. Your health journey will be no different.

Perhaps this is not the way we wish the world to be, but it's the way it is. I've fallen more times than I care to remember, and in truth I've often stayed down for a little longer than I should, yet there has always been a little voice in the back of my mind whispering:

"Never give up."

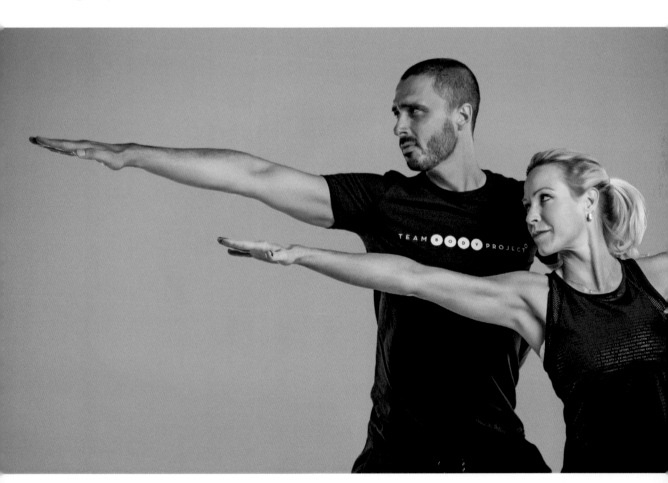

Sometimes I don't believe the voice. Sometimes I ask if it is speaking to me as I'm lying there feeling every inch the quitter. Yet the voice is always right. I don't quit, because if the philosophy of 'not giving up' is infused in your DNA, you will always get back up and carry on.

- You don't quit if you get knocked down on the way to your goal. Everybody gets knocked down.
- You don't quit if you get knocked down and take time to recover. Sometimes we need a rest.
- You only quit once you allow the punches of life to stop you from trying.

I'm not a great believer in mantras, yet this is one I have:

"Never give up."

We can choose to infuse this belief into our DNA and make it part of our story, or we can allow a different message to creep inside the story we tell ourselves, with an entirely different ending.

"I always quit."

'I always quit' becomes the default position of the human mind if we don't teach ourselves that it is false.

So start infusing a different message into your subconscious.

"Never give up."

"Never give up."

"NEVER give up."

If you can plant these four words inside your mind and allow them to spread and seep into every sinew of your body, you can achieve anything you want.

Three simple words that can change your life.

HOLD THE LINE
– CORE HABIT 5

On some days, you will not feel like exercising, and worse yet, some days you won't even feel motivated afterwards. Rather than a ray of sunlight shining on you at the end of a workout, you'll look up and see a black cloud in the sky, ready to pour its dirty rain on a musicless parade that nobody turned up to.

You will say, "I thought exercise was meant to make me feel better?"

On these days you may read posts of motivation and fanfare from other people and start to wonder whether exercise really is something for you.

I can assure you exercise is for you with just as much certainty as I can assure you that you will find days and even weeks like these.

So what should you do in these times?

Don't worry about pushing forwards and making great leaps of progress, just hold the line. Holding the line is just getting it done. No more.

Stand strong and tell the irresistible force that is trying to stop you from making progress that today you are an immovable object. You may not move forwards on days like these but you sure ain't letting it win!

Hold the line for the motivated and inspired version of you that is waiting behind the line, ready to crash through when the time is right. On these days, a huge victory is won as you trudge through the workout with less energy than a tortoise who took a sleeping pill after a carb-packed Christmas dinner.

That's holding the line in exercise terms! That is winning! The motivated and inspired you will thank you for holding the line as they burst through the line…and they will burst through the line sooner than you think!

Case study – Matthew, 62

In the past I would start an exercise plan and motor through for weeks, until one day, I no longer felt like exercising.

From nowhere I would always lose motivation. Even after a workout I would still feel flat. I thought there was something wrong with me so I would give up!

This time, rather than judge myself when I feel flat, I pick a lighter workout and just go through the motions. Feeling good just for holding it together.

This is the one difference and why I am now a fully committed lifetime exerciser.

INTRODUCTION TO EMOTIONAL EATING

Would thunder be half as majestic without lightning to illuminate the night sky with every roar?

Would Ginger Rogers float with such impossible elegance without the accomplished hands of Fred Astaire to guide her?

If they'd never met on a cold and dreary morning in 1950s Liverpool, would Lennon or McCartney have penned some of the most memorable songs of the 20th century?

You see, some things just belong together. Drawn to one another with an irresistible, magnetic force, they are unquestionably better off as a couple.

Don't be fooled, however, into thinking that just because things are drawn together, that they are richer for finding one another.

Things didn't turn out so well for Bonnie and Clyde, and while Romeo and Juliet may be lauded in posterity, it's fair to say that were their chance encounter avoided, they would probably have lived long and happy lives instead of an ever so romantic but ultimately unsatisfying 'his' and 'hers' ending.

Which leads me onto the irrepressible relationship between emotions and large amounts of readily available, highly digestible, completely unsuitable food.

Emotions are wild, ravenous creatures that don't respond to reason or logic because emotions are hungry.

"Biology, smiology"

We have two good feet for walking. Two eyes for looking at things. A couple of ever so useful hands for picking up the things that we see. We've been given two ears for hearing things and a mouth for telling people what we've heard.

That all makes sense.

What doesn't make quite as much sense is why an irrepressible sensor runs directly from our tummy to our brain, rewarding processed food consumption with a super-sized portion of 'feel good for about 10 minutes'.

Why does junk food release serotonin and dopamine? (Hormones that make us feel temporarily better.)

A doctor of ancestral eating patterns will no doubt enlighten me, so I'll pre-empt below:

"When there was a food shortage in our 'hunter gatherer' days, it was very important we ate lots of food to survive. Food was in short supply, therefore our brains would reward us for eating high calorie, high energy foods."

I thus retort: "Blah, blah blah-de-blah..."

A dollop of happy hormones to reward us for tucking into a raw mammoth thigh in such plighted circumstances seems somewhat surplus to requirements when we're already preventing certain death!

Be that as it may, there is no escaping the fact that eating high calorie, high energy foods releases feel-good hormones, and when whoever created the human body created the human body, they didn't factor in Häagen-Dazs competing with Ben & Jerry's to create the most deliciously flavoured ice cream the world has ever seen.

Which brings me onto the emotion/eating relationship.

It is destructive, unhealthy and damaging. If Emotions was Eating's spouse, Eating would terminate the marriage, citing unreasonable behaviour from Emotions as indisputable ground for decree absolute.

A separation

Health and contentment are two entirely distinct battles.

Statement 1: Becoming healthy will not necessarily equate to you feeling happier. Although it will probably help.

Statement 2: Becoming happier will not necessarily equate to healthy behaviours. Although it will probably help.

I've used the term 'happy' to embarrassingly oversimplify and incompetently describe the concept of an absence of the incalculable variety of negative emotional issues the human psyche can experience.

In this context, I'm pretty convinced perpetual 'happiness' is an impossibility.

I like to compare an emotional life to painting the Forth of Firth Bridge, (a bridge in Scotland, famous for always being painted, such is its vast size). Just when you think you've finished and stand back to inspect the wonderful job you've done, you notice that an old part of the bridge is starting to show signs of wear and tear and you're back to work again.

Since the job of emotional management is an ongoing one, linking emotions with eating is a monstrously bad idea.

Many experts correctly ascertain that if you solve your emotional problems, you will stop emotional eating. This is, of course, almost entirely true.

The problem being that nobody, ever, has solved the puzzle of fixing emotions.

There is another word for emotional struggle and strife.

That word is *life*.

So, if you're willing to accept that you're pretty unlikely to solve the mystery of life anytime soon, it shouldn't take a great leap of faith to accept that you'll need to take a different strategy to overcome emotional eating.

When you feel bad. Don't eat. Ask yourself why you feel bad. Then feel bad.

When you feel happy. Don't eat. Ask yourself what made you happy. Then feel happy.

When you feel scared. Don't eat. Ask yourself why you are afraid. Then feel scared.

Emotions know the square root of nothing about food. They have VERY important messages to deliver but they haven't got a single clue when it comes to cuisine.

Our emotional eating handbook provides you with five very simple habits to implement and beat emotional eating.

Will achieving your health goals reconcile all of the emotional struggles you have? No, it won't, but you will feel more resilient and able to confront life's challenges.

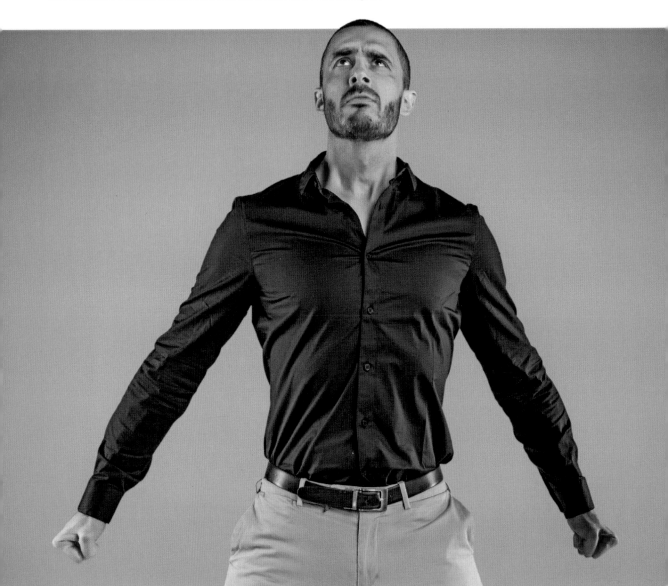

CONQUER EMOTIONAL EATING

Emotional eating has as much complexity as there are people in the world. Everybody has an entirely different experience.

On the other hand it is incredibly simple:

1. You eat impulsively and without thinking.
2. You eat for reasons beyond the need for food.
3. You hold false beliefs about food that prevent you from reaching your goals.

If we can remove the above three factors from the equation, we are left with only two times to eat:

1. When we are actually hungry.
2. When we have decided we are going to eat (including 'unhealthy' foods and celebrations).

With the five-step emotional eating plan we will give you five simple habits that, when implemented, will allow you to enjoy all types of food free from guilt and in quantities that are in line with your goals.

Physical hunger versus emotional appetite

It is important to separate the physiological need for food from the emotional appetite for it.

One is essential to survival and the other is a surefire way to ruin your goals!

Hunger is the physiological call to food	Appetite is the emotional call to food
Physical hunger builds up gradually	Emotional appetite comes on suddenly
Physical hunger is patient	Emotional appetite demands immediate attention
Physical hunger can be satisfied	Emotional appetite is insatiable
After eating for physical hunger you feel satisfied	After eating for emotional appetite you feel guilty
Physical hunger appears two to three hours after previous meal	Emotional appetite can appear at any time

The truth about hunger and weight loss

If you want to lose weight you will feel physiologically hungry and you won't always be able to satisfy it. The process of 'not having enough calories' is what will cause your body to raid the stores of fat to release them for energy.

If you want to make progress, you'll need to feel hungry from time to time. The difference with physiological hunger is after 30 minutes your body will free up stored fat for energy use and your hunger will pass.

Emotional appetite does not follow the same rules.

You are experiencing emotional appetite and driven to emotional eating any time you are not eating based on hunger signals. Emotional eating is never useful and this handbook will help you remove this habit and develop a healthy relationship with all foods.

The five habits

Action is the driver of all change.

We could write and talk about emotional eating all day, but only action creates change.

The emotional eating handbook has five proactive habits you can implement in order to create success.

Proactive habit 1 – write down your triggers

Actively try and highlight the moments you feel triggered to emotional eating.

- Is it boredom?
- Is it social events?
- Disappointment?
- Success?
- Fear?
- Anxiety?
- The smell of food?
- Relationships?
- Locations?

When it comes to behaviour, awareness is nine-tenths of the law. If you can successfully identify the triggers and moments that draw you towards emotional eating, you can start the process of overriding them and taking control of your decisions.

Your habit is to identify your triggers as they happen and create awareness.

Case study – Susan, 43

Susan was a lifetime emotional eater and despite exercising regularly and eating a healthy diet, her results were always hijacked by what she considered to be uncontrollable binge eating.

I asked her what caused the emotional eating. She thought she knew but I asked her to write down what those things were anyway.

The next week, she came back to see me and I asked her if she was happy to talk to me about what she had learned.

She was visibly shocked at how many different events and moments in her life were associated with food. While she had expected emotions like stress or anger to be triggers, the television, the phone ringing, her mum texting her, boredom and even walking past the bakers were triggering her.

Her entire life was littered with moments she had been hanging food on to 'cope' with.

In her words:

"When I actually asked myself if I was hungry or just being triggered by events, I was surprised at how easy it was to avoid emotional eating. Awareness was the key moment for me."

This was a revelation to Susan, and while it wasn't all plain sailing and hurdles were still to be leaped, from this point onwards we were finally able to help her reach her goals.

Proactive habit 2 – pause

The most valuable gift we can learn in mastery of self is the ability to pause and 'take a moment' before engaging in behaviour.

A profound pause that creates space for rationale.

Of all the habits we can create in defence of emotional eating this is the greatest of all.
While pausing for a single minute may seem such an insignificant amount of time, this moment creates a vast ocean between your emotions and your ultimate behaviour.

In the context of emotional eating that is groundbreaking.

In the newly formed ocean between you and your action, your logical mind can rise to the surface and enter the debate. (That is not to say your logical mind will always win the argument, but at least it will enter the conversation.)

Within this minute, a number of questions can arise.

"Do I really want that piece of cake? Maybe a handful of nuts is better?"

"Am I actually hungry? Maybe I'm bored?"

"How am I going to feel afterwards? Is it worth it?"

Work at developing this habit into your daily routine in the same way you work at exercising every day.

Here is the habit:

1. Whenever you are going to eat, set your phone/watch timer to 60 seconds.

2. In that 60 seconds, bring rationale to your decision. Ask yourself questions about your hunger:

- Am I hungry or thirsty?
- Am I hungry or am I trying to change the way I feel?
- Are there healthier options I could eat instead?
- What other things could I do instead?
- How does this decision align with my goals?
- Is this 'junk food' part of my plan or is it driven by emotions.
- What am I actually looking to achieve?
- Am I bored? Am I angry? Am I frustrated?

3. At the end of the 60 seconds, make the decision and take action accordingly.

4. If, five minutes later, you get driven to emotional eating again, repeat the process. Before ANY food passes your mouth; your behaviour is to pause for 60 seconds.

That is the proactive emotional eating habit you are introducing to your life.

Exercise ✓
Eat plenty of vegetables ✓
Drink water ✓
Pause for a minute before eating ✓

Creating habits is central to success. Take every habit you build seriously if you believe that habit is important to your long-term success.

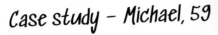
Case study – Michael, 59

Michael was a compulsive eater. When I asked him to write down what his triggers were he struggled to identify them, even a week later.

"I almost go into an out of body experience. I don't even know why I'm doing it or enjoy it most of the time. I just kinda do it and then think "oh no, what did I do that for?".

I gave him a specific habit to work on. Rather than ask what the trigger is, just pause before you are about to eat whatever it is you are about to eat.

This became the central habit Michael needed to break his emotional eating habit. He had a very clear set of goals and creating the habit of 'pausing' gave him time to bring his long-term goals to the conversation.

Michael is a slightly unique case, but not that unique amongst men I have worked with. They often find it harder to identify triggers but can be very effective at aligning goals with behaviours within a structure.

Proactive habit 3 – control your environment

If the foods you desire when confronting emotional eating are not available, then you can't have them. If healthier foods and/or water are available you will have them instead.

This strategy really is that simple.

There is a two-step approach to controlling your environment.

1. Remove all temptations

- Clear your cupboards of tempting foods, treats and snacks that you know you would be tempted by if available.
  (We know this can be hard with small children, but not impossible.)
- Remove temptations from your car and anywhere else you may go.
- Remove temptations from work as much as possible. (We understand this can be hard too.)
- Take minimum cash to places like the cinema or coffee shops, so you can only buy what you planned for and nothing more.

2. Have suitable replacements available at all times

- Make a list of healthy snacks you can enjoy (replacement snacks are a last resort).
- Have them available.
- Have a bottle of water available as a first solution all the time.

Note: *This habit should be seen as a temporary habit rather than a permanent one.*

Proactive habit 4 – create a new habit

There is a saying in behaviour change circles.

If an inanimate object can do it, it's not a behaviour. A chair can 'not eat' therefore, 'not eating' is not a behaviour.

If we are going to stop one behaviour, in this instance emotional eating, we need to replace it with another positive one.

What positive habits can you replace your emotional eating with?

- Drinking a glass of water?
- Taking five minutes of meditation?
- Walking 500 steps?
- Reading a book for five minutes?
- Doing 10 push ups?

Find a positive habit that you can enforce to replace your emotional eating habit and make that a habit.

If you are an emotional eater you must take this as seriously as you take your daily workout for your goals.

Note: As a last resort you can have a healthy snack as your replacement behaviour but this is a short-term solution. We are trying to avoid eating for emotions, so using food is not ideal.

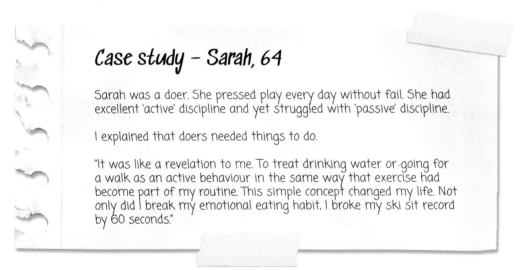

Case study – Sarah, 64

Sarah was a doer. She pressed play every day without fail. She had excellent 'active' discipline and yet struggled with 'passive' discipline.

I explained that doers needed things to do.

"It was like a revelation to me. To treat drinking water or going for a walk as an active behaviour in the same way that exercise had become part of my routine. This simple concept changed my life. Not only did I break my emotional eating habit, I broke my ski sit record by 60 seconds."

P.S. In case you hadn't guessed Sarah had decided to do the ski sit whenever she was caught up in emotional appetite.

Proactive habit 5 – think sustainable

Feeling restricted and deprived of foods is not positive for long-term goals. Many people are frightened to eat foods that have always been associated with comfort eating, but it is important to change your relationship with food if you want long-term success.

Provided you have a predominantly healthy diet, there will be no considerable difference to your diet between choosing a banana or a small chocolate bar or cookie as a snack.

Having reasonably sized snacks that you enjoy scheduled into your plan – those you have previously overeaten and felt guilty eating in periods of emotional eating – will change your relationships with these foods to a positive and enjoyable one.

No food is good or bad. It is just food.

You can have a balanced and enjoyable relationship with all types of food, provided you either:

A. Have them scheduled into a nutrition plan that is based around your goals.
B. Eat when you are physiologically hungry.
C. Do not eat when you are emotionally hungry.

Case study – Ali, 37

Friday evening came around and Ali had enjoyed a really great week of healthy eating and exercising.

She took a look in the cupboards and saw a big bag of Doritos.

"I felt I deserved a treat for all of my hard work in the week. I opened the bag, intending only to have a few, but ended up eating the whole bag. I felt guilty afterwards and felt like I'd ruined all of my hard work."

I spoke with Ali the next day and explained that one bag of Doritos would have negligible impact on her overall results and to let it go and not turn an insignificant moment into a disaster.

I then explained the importance of having snacks and treats built into the week so you can prepare, plan and ultimately change your relationship with food.

We agreed that Ali could have a portion of Doritos every Friday night with a glass of wine to relax, enjoy and celebrate her accomplishments. Rather than feel guilty, Ali enjoyed her Doritos and developed a positive relationship with what had previously been a comfort food.

For as long as I worked with Ali she retained this habit and looked forwards to her weekly treat while achieving her long-term goals.

Final word

These habits are not ideas.
These habits are not concepts.
These habits are not words for you to read and agree with.

They are habits – like exercise or eating vegetables.

THE FIVE HABITS

Habit 1 – Write down your triggers

Habit 2 – Pause

Habit 3 – Control your environment

Habit 4 – Create a new habit

Habit 5 – Think sustainable

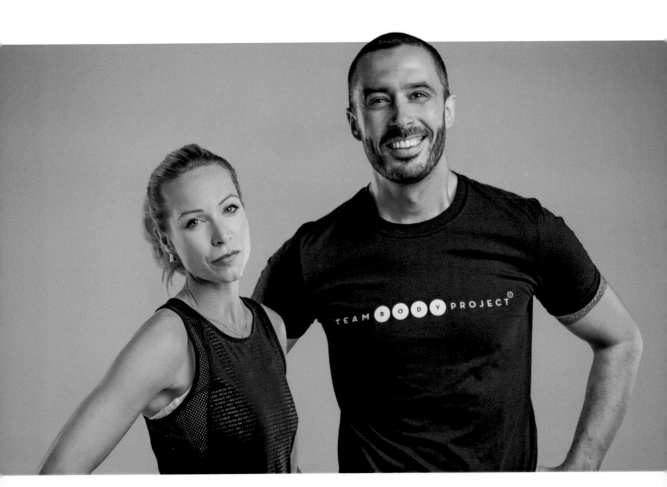

HEALTHY FOOD THOUGHTS

To develop a healthy relationship with foods, rather than an emotional one, it is helpful to have a list of healthy thoughts around food.

Print this out and place it on your fridge or somewhere else you look every day.

HEALTHY FOOD THOUGHTS

1.   Food is just food.
Food is not anything except food. It is not the reason for my problems, nor is it the solution to them. It is just food.

2.   Eating for social reasons is great.
I eat healthily for many reasons. This does not mean enjoying foods of all types with friends and family is not a good thing, provided it is part of my plan and in line with my goals.

3.   If I want results I can't just 'eat what I want'.
Everything worth having in life requires some form of compromise. A healthy body requires me to consider the foods I eat. A healthy body and life is more valuable to me than food.

4.   Habits are the driving force behind my ultimate results.
It is the habits I implement on a daily basis that will create the healthy body I want to have.

5.   If I make a mistake it doesn't make too much long-term difference.
I am not perfect. Sometimes I make a mistake and don't stay with my plan. That is fine as long as I let it go and move on.

6.   Food doesn't solve my stress or make things better.
I understand that food has never solved any of the problems in my life, but I do not blame it for any of the problems I have either. It is just food.

7.   Healthy eating doesn't mean perfect eating.
I can eat between 70% and 90% healthy foods and still have a healthy body. No food is bad or good. It is just food.

8.   Eating less or more of something is my choice.
I do not 'have' to eat fewer calories or lose weight. I choose to eat fewer calories and more vegetables because a healthy body is important to me.

9.   Food helps me achieve my goals.
Healthy nutrition makes me feel better, perform better and achieve all my goals in life better.

10.   My body is valuable to me. It deserves good fuel.
I value my body as the most valuable asset I will ever own. I will respect it and give it the fuel it deserves.

RECAP

Five core habits – one objective: Achieving your goals

Practise these habits as rigorously and with as much dedication as you apply to your workouts and there is only one outcome.

Success.

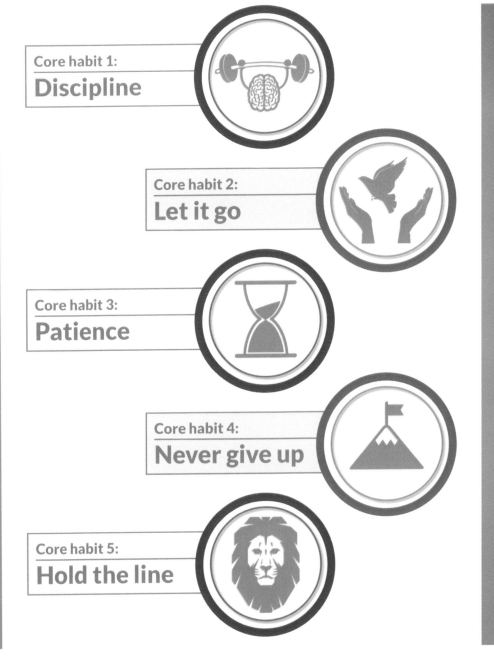

Core habit 1:
Discipline

Core habit 2:
Let it go

Core habit 3:
Patience

Core habit 4:
Never give up

Core habit 5:
Hold the line

If you can combine these core habits with **Harry's Habits**, the world is your oyster.

Harry's Habits

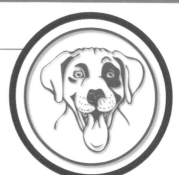

Harry wishes you every success as you Transform for Life.

And he'd like you to know that dropping food at the dinner table is more than acceptable.

- Make healthy habits non-negotiable
- Focus on a permanent lifestyle change
- Question false beliefs
- Don't compare yourself to others
- Be kind to yourself
- Celebrate every victory

Now you know *The Science*.

You understand *The Art of Change*.

It's time to *Transform for Life* and develop *The Blueprint*.

TEAM NSV (NON-SCALE VICTORY)

Team NSV

Name: Jo Osman
Location: Singapore
Age: 46
Favourite workout: Championship Boxing 2
Time with team: 3 months

"I wish I had understood how powerful the NSV would be on this journey. Numbers no longer rule my life or dictate my motivation or self-worth and since I have stopped using the scale as my oracle the benefits I have achieved both mentally and physically are immensely satisfying, however small."

The non-scale victory is something we designed to ensure focus on the more regular benefits of health 'beyond the scale'.

A non-scale victory is any successful progress you have made beyond your aesthetic goals.

These non-scale victories are crucial to our long-term success as they allow us to focus on the reasons we are exercising and eating healthily beyond our aesthetic goals.

This is important for two reasons:

1. They are powerful motivators when the scale or measuring tape doesn't budge.
2. You will develop a plethora of reasons to keep exercising and eating healthily after you have reached your goals.

Examples of members' NSVs:

Team NSV

Name: Mike Starnes
Location: Reading, UK
Age: 33
Favourite workout: Interval coaching
Time with team: 9 months

"Outlasting Daniel on the ski sits…"

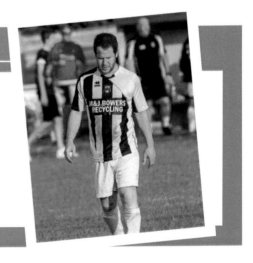

Team NSV

Name: Kay Esmond
Location: Queensland, Australia
Age: 36
Favourite workout: Sparta
Time with team: 11 months

"Bought a medium size dress online for my stepson's formal...and it's too big! So I'm off to get a small!"

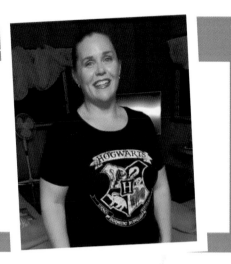

Team NSV

Name: Emily Richards
Location: Utah, USA
Age: 31
Favourite workout: Spit and Sawdust
Time with team: 7 months

"My non-scale victory is overcoming the belief that making one (or two, or ten) health mistakes (like eating a whole cake or something...) doesn't mean I might as well give up now. Just because I went ten days without exercising doesn't mean I might as well go eleven. It's definitely a mental non-scale victory!"

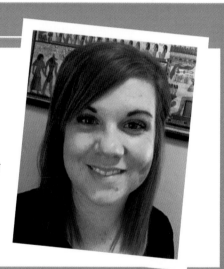

Team NSV

Name: Shundranique Gordon King
Location: Alabama, USA
Age: 33
Favourite workout: Interval Cardio
Time with team: 36 months

"All of the 'you look so good,' 'keep doing what you're doing' compliments I've been getting lately."

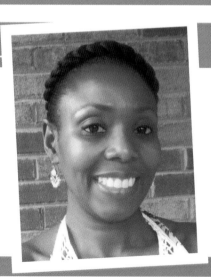

Team NSV

Name: Lisamaria Collaco
Location: Saint Louis, USA
Age: 35
Favourite workout: Still Personal
Time with team: 18 months

"Being here today after a severe bout of depression. TBP helped me to heal and recover."

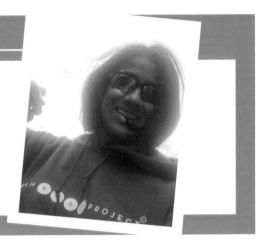

Team NSV

Name: Anita Hatters
Location: Australia
Age: 30
Favourite workout: Superhero Intense
Time with team: 18 months

"Arm and shoulder muscles are appearing (even under my skin!!)"

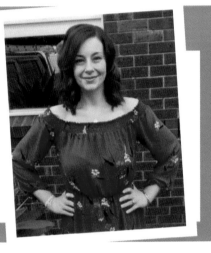

THE
BLUEPRINT

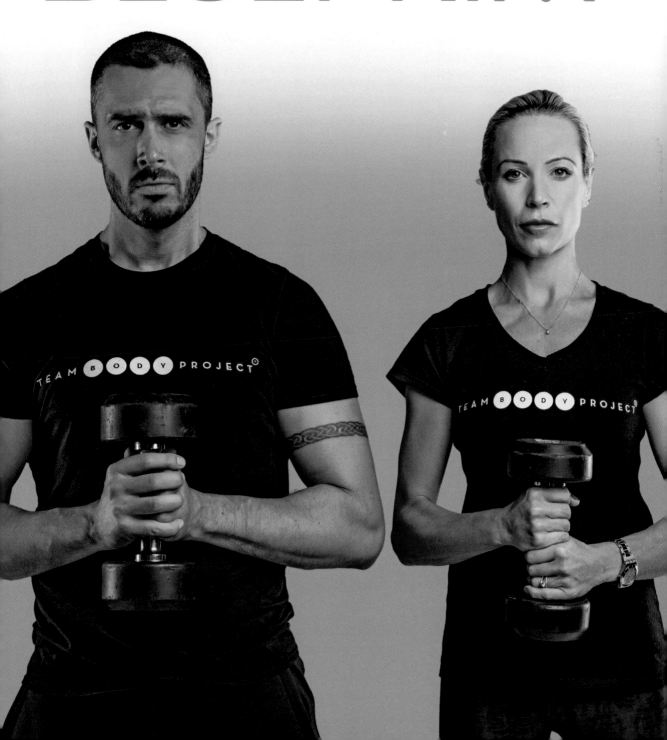

INTRODUCTION TO THE BLUEPRINT

Important: Read before starting your Blueprint

If you have read *The Science of Physical Transformation* and *The Art of Change* there is a good possibility you are already feeling overwhelmed with the information.

If you haven't read the *The Science of Physical Transformation* and *The Art of Change*, *The Blueprint* is probably about to overwhelm you.

The purpose of *Transform for Life* is to leave you in no doubt concerning the mechanisms behind physical change. This is not a an oversimplified 'diet' book, it is a scientific process of monitoring and producing predictable physical change.

Many people feel frustrated that they *"Can't lose the last few pounds"* or feel confused as to why, whatever they seem to do, they just can't lose weight.

Transform for Life strips away uncertainty and doubt surrounding physical change.

Having helped people make physical changes for most of my adult life, everything I have learned is available for you to apply in this book.

However, knowing what to do to change your body does not mean you have to follow through with it. You no longer need to be victim to an ever changing diet industry - you can shake off the shackles of confusion and replace them with pillars of knowledge.

What you do with them, is up to you.

Transform for Life empowers you to make informed decisions based on facts. It does not suggest you should do anything.

Carefully consider the following points before you decide on your approach to your health plan:

If you want to be happy, healthy and fit - accepting of yourself and your body - reading *The Science of Physical Transformation* and *The Art of Change* alongside implementing *The Quickstart Guide* will be an excellent route.

You will be able to make better overall decisions based on the knowledge you have learned, making small tweaks along the way.

On the other hand, if you are determined to achieve the body you want, driven by a certainty that you want to lose the pounds and/or achieve the body shape you desire, *The Blueprint* will get you there. If you do choose to follow *The Blueprint*, be prepared. This is not a simple, quick fix method.

It requires work, patience and plenty of frustration en route. Every client I ever coached presented entirely unique challenges, and you will face your own.

You will possibly feel overwhelmed, overstretched and, in the early stages, completely out of your comfort zone.

Genuine change doesn't happen through doing the things we have always done, or by living inside of our comfort zone, within a safety net of behaviours we are used to. Lifelong change exists beyond the familiar and in a world where everything feels strange and new. Open your mind to the challenge in front of you and your results will be beyond expectations.

Nothing makes me happier than seeing an individual make *the break* into new comfort zones and enjoying the rewards that come with it.

How to use this section

The Blueprint will help you set a starting point and a strong foundation for your health plan.

- Setting goals: Here you will define the reasons for taking part (pages 151-154)
- Fitness test (optional): This will help you decide on which workout plan to follow (Page 156) **Blueprint task 1**
- Choose a workout plan: Select a workout plan suitable for your goals and current fitness (pages 157-158) **Blueprint task 2**
- Setting NEAT: Make decisions around daily activity (pages 159-160) **Blueprint task 3**
- Starting calories: Decide on calorie intake (pages 161-167) **Blueprint task 4**
- Healthy eating ratios: Decide how much of your diet you choose to be healthy (Pages 168 - 171) **Blueprint task 5**
- FLUX: Decide how you will flux calories to improve body composition and performance (Page 172-177) **Blueprint task 6**
- Macronutrient ratios: Decide on your ratios of protein, carbs and fats (pages 178-181) **Blueprint task 7**
- Tracking: Here you will learn how to track and monitor your progress (pages 182-191)
- Measurements: Here you will set a benchmark to measure yourself against (Pages 193-194) **Blueprint task 8**
- Getting equipped: Here we will make sure you have everything you need to succeed (pages 195-196)
- Finalising your Blueprint and Blueprint light: (Pages 197-200)

What is the right option for you?

There are three ways of using the information in *Transform for Life*:

The Blueprint	A comprehensive approach to lifetime health
The Blueprint Light	Options within The Blueprint which provide a less overwhelming approach to lifetime health
The Quickstart	To help you get going immediately. You will find this in *Additional Resources*.

Before you decide on which one you want to follow, I want to ask two questions that can support any decisions you make.

Question 1: Has what you have done in the past worked in the way that you have wanted it to?

This is not the same as short-term weight loss. These are fundamental health changes that you can be confident will stay with you for life.

You may have preconceived ideas about what you need to do to achieve lifetime health:

- This is too much work
- Checking details would make me feel anxious
- Tracking calories is obsessive
- I don't need to spend that much time on health, all I need to do is workout
- I just need to eat less, I've done it before

If you want a different outcome, you may need a different approach and to let go of preconceived ideas that have not supported permanent change.

When approached correctly, *Transform for Life* is a process of learning how your body responds to food, exercise and activity.

Question 2: How important is achieving your weight management goals to you?

If achieving a physical goal and keeping it is 10/10 on your importance scale, spending additional time and effort for the next several weeks on learning and developing a tailored approach is certainly well worth it.

If it is quite important to you, but not worth the extra effort, choosing *The Quickstart Guide* would be a better option.

Aligning expectation with effort is crucial for perpetual engagement.

Choosing an approach

If you use *The Quickstart Guide* and don't get results, you can always change. Likewise, if you choose *The Blueprint* but find it too much, you can always revert to a less time-consuming process.

Provided you line up your choice against your expectations you can be proud of yourself and the outcome.

Method 1: The Blueprint

The Blueprint is the coaching system I used with professional athletes, people who want to make permanent change, long-term dieters who can't break lifelong habits and anybody who wants a guarantee that effort would be equalled by outcome.

This is not a restrictive plan, it is a comprehensive one. It is comprehensive so we can avoid the pitfalls, obsessive behaviours and downfalls of simpler health plans.

Thorough is paying attention to the details. We want this.
Obsession is becoming consumed by them. We do not want this.

During *The Blueprint* you will still be able to:

- Eat foods you enjoy
- Not feel overly restricted
- Exercise for an amount of time that works for you
- Live a balanced and healthy life

The Blueprint is as restrictive, enjoyable and relevant as you choose to make it.

The Blueprint is suitable for those who:

- Want to create a blueprint that is perfect for them
- Want a health plan they can follow for life
- Are willing to put the time and effort in to learn about their body
- Are determined to put the dieting cycle behind them for good

We do not expect you to spend the rest of your life tracking food and exercise and analysing your behaviours and habits, even if you are following *The Blueprint*.

The time you put into understanding your body and habits will enable you to create a personal *Health Blueprint* that will last for the rest of your life.

Your first week will help you set the foundations for a nutrition and exercise plan that you can follow in the long-term.

Note: *As you move through the chapters you will be given tasks to complete in* **Your Health Blueprint.**

Method 2: The Blueprint Light

The Blueprint Light introduces you to focused health in a less overwhelming way than *The Blueprint* by offering you 'light' options as you move through the chapter.

Tracking is introduced to raise awareness, but at a far simpler level than *The Blueprint:*

- Follow our workout plans
- Learn how to track your intake without the pressure of meeting targets
- Learn alternative forms of tracking
- Make changes based on what you feel comfortable with

This method will raise awareness around intake and *cause and effect* without the pressure that can be associated with meeting targets. Often a short period following *The Blueprint Light* makes people feel more comfortable moving on to *The Blueprint*.

The Blueprint Light is suitable for those who:

- Want to make permenant changes but feel overwhelmed at the thought of *The Blueprint*
- Are new to exercise and nutrition
- Feel ready to make changes but want to do it at their own pace.

Note: *As you move through the chapters you will be given tasks to complete in* **Your Health Blueprint Light.**

Method 3: The Quickstart (pages 259-266)

The idea behind *The Quickstart* is simple and, for all the detailed science and precision of this book, this method can be remarkably effective

- Follow our workout plans
- Try and eat healthy foods more often and processed foods less
- If you want to lose weight, try to think about how much you eat and do more NEAT.

The Quickstart is suitable for those who:

- Don't have the time or inclination to track
- Want a simple health routine to slip into their lives
- Are new to exercise and healthy eating

Many thousands of people have followed this advice and achieved everything they want and more.

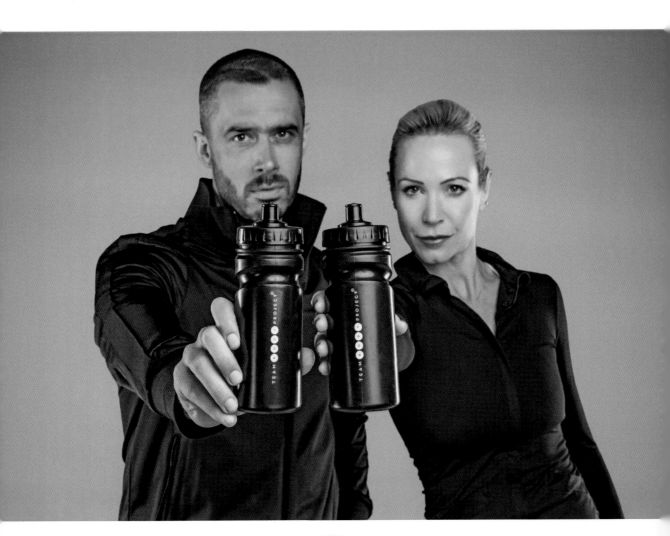

SETTING YOUR GOALS

Write your goals down here:

GOALS

Note: *You may wish to come back to this after you have taken your measurements.*

WHY?

What are the motivators that will keep you on track?

Why you are taking part in *Transform for Life*? When the going gets tough, which it will, you need to understand what drove you to start in the first place:

- Your specific physical goals
- The positive impacts on your life from achieving your targets and expectations
- The negative impacts on your life if they don't happen

After you have completed the tasks on this page, when the going gets tough this is a good page to return to and remind you of why you started in the first place.

Goals

What are your physical, aesthetic and performance goals?

1. Make sure your goals are measurable and specific.
   Example: if you don't have body fat calipers, you can't measure fat loss, so bodyweight and measurements are better.

2. Make sure your goals are realistic and achievable.
   Example: you can target up to 2 lb (0.9 kg) of weight loss a week and up to 0.5 lb (0.2 kg) of muscle gain a week (not simultaneously). If you have 100 lb (45 kg) you want to lose, this can not be healthily achieved in less than 12 months.

The Five Whys technique

If you struggle to reveal what your motivators are, the Five Whys technique is a very useful method of discovery. Ask yourself 'why?' until you reach the true conclusion.

Here's an example:

What is your goal?

1. I want to lose weight
   – Why do you want to lose weight?
2. So I have more energy
   – Why do you want to have more energy?
3. So I can run around the park with my children
   – Why do you want to run around the park with your children?
4. My relationship with them is the most important thing in the world to me, and I want them to see me as healthy
   – Why do you want them to see you as healthy?
5. So they are influenced to live healthy lives of their own.

Example case study:

Goals

Lose 40 lb in 12 months

Get back into my pre-baby clothes

Run a 5 km with my husband

Do a 90 second plank

Question 1: What negative impact does not being at your goal have on your life?

Why I want to achieve my goals

I hate going on holiday and worrying about the way I look rather than spending time with my family.

My mum had a heart attack at 55 and i'm terrified of the same thing happening to me.

I can't spend any more of my life thinking about and worrying about my weight.

Question 2: What are the top reasons why you want to meet your goals and enjoy the health benefits that accompany them?

Why I want to achieve my goals

I want my children to see me as a positive example of health and make healthy decisions themselves.

I want to be able to choose clothes i want to wear and feel good in my body.

I want to be active, healthy and live a long life.

Discovering why

The following two questions are designed to help you uncover your true motivators for success. If you have set a goal, it is because you would prefer to be there, than where you are at the moment.

Question 1: What negative impact does not being at your goal have on your life?

Some people are driven by the carrot and some by the stick. The negative impact of not achieving goals can be more compelling than the positive impact of achieving them. Why is it important to not fail at achieving your goals?

Consider any negative impacts of not achieving your goals and write them in the box on the next page.

Why I want to achieve my goals

Question 2: What are the top reasons why you want to meet your goals and enjoy the health benefits that accompany them?

Remember to keep asking 'why?' until you are satisfied with your core motivation.

Consider any positive impacts of achieving your goals and write them in the box below.

Why I want to achieve my goals

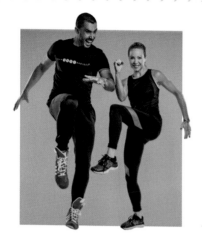

The Blueprint is the most advanced and detailed blueprint you can create.

If you wish to create a less time consuming and overwhelming blueprint, you can use the **The Blueprint Light** options provided. You will find the *Blueprint Light* tasks in the light blue boxes throughout the text.

If you wish to get going as quickly as possible, please refer to **The Quickstart Guide** in *Additional Resources*.

GETTING STARTED

Choosing the right exercise plan that works for you and fits around your lifestyle is crucial for long-term success. Before you follow the guidelines below and take the fitness test and/or select a suitable workout plan, consider the following:

Long-term exercise commitment

Although it is acceptable and even encouraged to spend periods of time doing additional exercise (we call them 'accelerators' – *Turbos* and *Sculptors*) for now, focus on your long-term, sustainable exercise routine.

- The first intention is to build a baseline habit
- Your daily workout is a baseline habit, so create a habit you can sustain
- Additional exercise is an accelerator
- Once you have established your baseline then you can add 'results-focused accelerators'

TASK

Think hard. Decide how much exercise you can do daily in the **long-term** and how many times a week.

This module will help you choose the initial exercise plan for you to follow. Once you have chosen your plan you can schedule the workouts in your calendar.

Compliance reminder

- The first rule of exercise is compliance
- The second rule of exercise is compliance
- The third rule of exercise is compliance

Nothing is more important in your long-term health success than 'Getting it done'. You can track exercise compliance using *The Exercise Compliance Tracker* (Page 256) located in the *Additional Resources* section.

THE FITNESS TEST

Before you start following a *Team Body Project* workout program we recommend finding your starting point. We've designed a fitness test that assesses various aspects of fitness using a few standard exercises.

1. Upper body strength – press up (moderated or full)
2. Lower body strength – squat and ski sit
3. Core strength – plank (moderated or full) and sit up
4. Cardio fitness – burpee (moderated or full)

Guidance only: This fitness score should be seen as a guide only. Given the limited amount of exercises, in which some of you may be particularly strong or weak, it is not definitive.

Why a fitness test?

1. Most people are stronger in certain areas. This test will enable them to highlight areas for development.
2. The fitness test provides you with a benchmark to track your progress. As you move through our programs it's exciting to track how far you've come.
3. Taking the fitness test will allow us to suggest the most suitable Team Body Project workout program for you.

Opting out of the fitness test

You may decide that the fitness test contains exercises you don't like or can't do. Perhaps you don't feel ready for the fitness test or you are confident in your own ability.

If you are not ready to take the fitness test we suggest you start with either:

- The Development Plan
- The Trainee Plan

If you are not taking the fitness test but are confident in your own fitness levels you can read the guidelines for each of the following workout programs to decide on which program to follow.

Take the fitness test now before returning to this module:

www.teambodyproject.com/fitness-test

What happens after the fitness test?

Once the fitness test is complete we will recommend a workout plan based on your score. Guidelines on suitable fitness test scores are in this module for all exercise plans.

TASK 1: THE FITNESS TEST

Note your fitness test score on Your *Health Blueprint* (page 199) or Your *Health Blueprint Light* (page 200) .

CHOOSING A WORKOUT PROGRAM

Workout with Team Body Project

Working out with Team Body Project makes exercise simple. You can workout from the comfort of your own home while achieving everything you need to with your body.

Once you have chosen a workout program with Team Body Project, the guesswork is taken away. All you have to do is follow the plan and mark the workouts as complete – we'll guide you every step of the way.

You'll be covered for resistance training, cardio, pilates and mobilisation and your progress will be continuous.

Follow the link below to choose a suitable exercise program for your current fitness levels and goals. You can create a free account with team body project by visiting:

www.teambodyproject.com

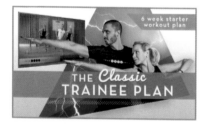
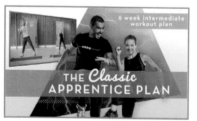
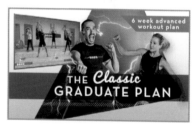

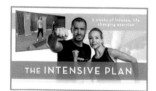
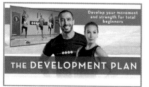
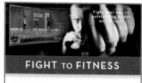
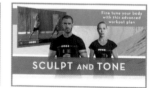

Other methods of exercise

If you choose not to work out with Team Body Project you can still set yourself an exercise program in a number of ways.

1. You can join a gym. The instructors at the gym will set you a suitable exercise routine and you can take part in the group classes.
2. You can start running or cycling. Many people find this to be an effective method of exercising.
3. You can take up an athletic sport like squash, football or badminton.
4. You can start swimming, rowing or taking part in other water sports.

Many methods of exercise are available and choosing the one that is right for you is important. All safe exercise is good exercise. The 'best' exercise for you is the method that works for you. Team Body Project workout plans are comprehensive, progressive and effective. They are also designed for convenience and ease of use - but if you don't enjoy them, please do find something else. We won't be offended. I promise!

TASK 2: CHOOSE A WORKOUT PLAN

Add your chosen workout plan to Your *Health Blueprint* (page 199) or Your *Health Blueprint Light* (page 200).

Lily's Laws

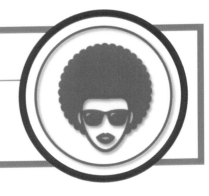

- Exercise to stimulate muscle growth and fat loss

Well done. You have taken care of a law of change.

SETTING NEAT

Non-Exercise Activity Thermogenesis (NEAT) is activity beyond your focused exercise and natural metabolism. It's a combination of your normal daily activity, your posture and your general movement – anything that uses energy beyond deliberate exercise and your baseline metabolic rate (BMR).

NEAT matters a lot. How many steps you walk, what you do when the adverts come on the television, whether you take the stairs or the lift, how you fill your break times at work, what activities you do with the kids, how much you fidget, what you do when your train is running late… these are all examples of NEAT.

Ignoring NEAT has a far greater impact on your metabolism than anything else.

- Buy a tracker
- Make good choices
- Be active

Moderate versus Low NEAT over 12 weeks

	Person 1: Moderate NEAT	Person 2: Low NEAT
NEAT	+500 kcal per day	+250 kcal per day
Calorie intake	1,500 kcal	1,500 kcal
Exercise	30 minutes = 250 kcal	30 minutes = 250 kcal
Weekly difference	1,750 kcal more burned than Person 2	1,750 kcal less burned than Person 1
12 week weight difference	Lost 6 lb more than person 2*	Lost 6 lb less than person 1*

*assuming 3,500 kcal = 1 lb in bodyweight

Deciding on NEAT

The main way we control NEAT is by tracking our steps. The majority of phones have free apps to use or you can buy an activity tracker.

NEAT table

Low NEAT: Less than < 5,000 steps per day
Moderate NEAT: 5,000 – 10,000 steps per day
Higher NEAT: More than > 10,000 steps per day

TASK 3: THE IMPORTANCE OF NEAT

Add your chosen NEAT steps per day to Your *Health Blueprint* (page 199) or Your *Health Blueprint Light* (page 200).

Lily's Laws

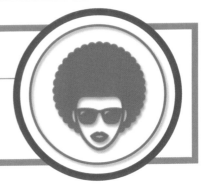

- NEAT is an important aspect of your metabolic rate

Well done. You have taken care of another law of change.

Additional exercise support

To learn more about exercise, including modifications, resistance training, rest periods and how to use *Turbos and Sculptors*, you can read *The Exercise Handbook* in *Additional Resources*.

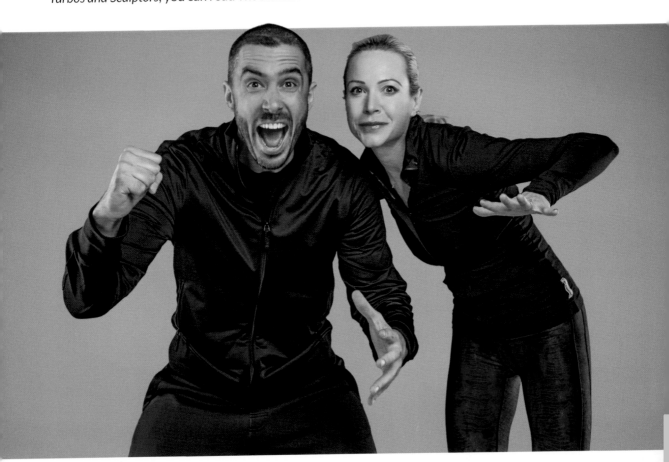

GETTING STARTED WITH NUTRITION

With the help of Lily's Laws, we are going to ensure every aspect of your nutrition is considered to ensure the best possible long-term results for you.

Lily's Laws

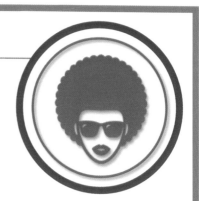

Lily wanted to pop by to remind us that nutrition is a vital component to change.

- Calorie balance
- Anabolic and catabolic flux
- Sufficient carbohydrates
- Sufficient protein
- Sufficient fat
- Drink enough water
- Eat plenty of vegetables
- Limit processed food intake

STARTING CALORIES

IMPORTANT

1. Setting your starting calories is something that should not cause you stress.
2. Meeting your calorie targets is something that should not cause you stress.

If setting calories, meeting calorie targets and tracking calories does make you feel stressed in any way, please consider following the *QuickStart guide*, using our *intuitive eating guidelines* or trying *The Blueprint light* suggestions for a few weeks.

Starting calories

Your starting calories are not nearly as important as the changes and adaptations you make over the coming weeks, based on the data you gather.

Many people spend hours worrying about the amount of calories they should start with and whether the quantity is too high or too low.

Every calorie calculator will provide you with a different guideline and none is necessarily correct or incorrect. It is impossible for any calculator or equation to know what the correct starting point for maximum fat loss and muscle retention for you is.

The calorie starting point you choose is unlikely to be exactly correct. Only through the process of tracking will you know how many calories cause you to lose fat/build muscle/stay the same.

Based on your results over the coming weeks and months, you will adjust your calories and every aspect of your *Blueprint* until you find your own personal goldilocks zone.

Using the Transform for Life Calculations for calories

If you used the MyFitnessPal* algorithm it would almost certainly give you a much lower starting point than the guidelines we provide here in *The Blueprint*.

Many people are surprised at how high our calorie recommendations are. At Team Body Project we are conservative with calorie reductions for the following reasons:

1. Our goal is for you to eat higher calories whilst losing FAT.

Not to lose WEIGHT as fast as possible and potentially dropping muscle.

If you have a small calorie deficit created through food consumption and a further calorie deficit through exercise, this maximises fat loss and encourages muscle retention.

2. If you go straight to (example) 1200 kcal per day, further reductions are impossible when you hit a plateau.

If you are eating 1700 kcal and losing 1 lb a week, you may not be losing weight as fast as on a lower calorie diet but:

- If you stop losing weight you can still reduce calories.
- You are certainly losing a very high percentage of fat (and you may be building muscle).
- You will have more energy and train better.
- You will feel less deprived.
- You are more likely to keep on track.

If you are eating 1200 kcal and losing 2lb a week:

- If you stop losing weight you can't reduce calories any further.
- You could well be losing some muscle (and will certainly not be building new muscle).
- You will have less energy and struggle to train.
- You may feel constantly hungry, irritable.
- You are less likely to keep on track.

So, rather than worry about your starting calories being too high, too low or anything in between, be confident that whatever your starting calories are, they will provide you with valuable feedback that you can adapt based on your goals.

A. If you gain a pound and train well?
Congratulations, you've just gained a pound of muscle that will help you in your journey.
You know what it takes for you to build muscle.

B. If you stay the same weight?
Congratulations, you know what your calorie balance is.

C. If you lose a pound and you want to?
Congratulations, you've nailed it.

D. If you lose 3 pounds?
Congratulations, you can now eat more food and still lose weight.

Using the Blueprint guidelines alongside activity trackers and MyFitnessPal

If you are going to follow our guidelines while using activity trackers and the MyFitnessPal application, it is important you turn off the automatic settings in MyFitnessPal and set to manual.

This way MyFitnessPal will not adjust your calories based on your activity levels. You can still enter your workouts and data into the MyFitnessPal application, but they will not affect the recommended calories and macronutrients you have set yourself.

On flux days you don't need to change the settings, you simply need to increase your intake according to your flux calculations (more details in section on setting flux)

MyFitnessPal is a sophisticated online calorie tracker we suggest using if you wish to track calories. We have free guidelines on how to use MyFitnessPal if you follow this link:

www.teambodyproject.com/additional-resources

Using MyFitnessPal recommendations

If you use set up MyFitnessPal in conjunction with a fitness tracker, like fitbit, it will adjust your required calories based on your activity levels. Therefore, if you are using an activity tracker synced with MyFitnessPal, you should not enter any exercise that the activity tracker is able to monitor.

Don't enter things like walking or running, Team Body Project workouts, or anything else that requires lots of body movement.

If you enter these exercises, you could double the calorie burn, which will result in you thinking you can consume more calories.

If you decide to use the MyFitnessPal algorithms and automatic activity information, MyFitnessPal will make adjustments to your calories based on your activity levels.

Pros of using MyFitnessPal automatic recommendations

- Much less work for you when the process is automated.
- You always adjust calories based on what you are doing and therefore don't risk eating too few calories.

Cons of using MyFitnessPal automatic recommendations

- You are not learning about how your body is working and tuning in to the signals - you are just responding to automated recommendations.
- Your calorie levels are always tracking at the same deficit against your baseline.
- You need to adjust the settings when you choose to introduce a flux day. (more details in section on setting flux)

Calorie tracking is not just for weight loss

If you 'just' want to lose a bit of weight and be a little healthier, follow *The Quickstart guide* confidently and happily.

Expectations drive everything. What are your expectations?

If you expect a specific outcome you must follow a specific plan. Whether that outcome is results based or sustainability based, the same rules apply.

If you want and expect to be exercising for the rest of your life, *The Blueprint* will help you achieve this.

If you want and expect to look a certain way or achieve a certain weight, *The Blueprint* will help you do this.

The Blueprint is designed to maximise fat loss, muscle retention and metabolic rate.

The Blueprint is designed to sculpt your body shape, improve your muscle tone and develop your performance.

The Blueprint is designed to develop a plan that works for you, for life.

You can lose a few pounds and get healthy with *The Quickstart guide*

You wouldn't waste money hiring a personal trainer if you just wanted to "lose a few pounds" because that's easily achievable with a little exercise and slightly fewer calories.

You'd hire a Personal Trainer if you wanted to maximise your physique, performance and long term outcome.

The same principle should apply to the time and effort you apply to *The Blueprint*.

The Blueprint is designed to:

- Find a long term health plan that works for you; especially if you have a history of yo-yo dieting
- Maximise fat loss when losing weight
- Minimise muscle loss when losing weight
- Maintain high performance and energy
- Maintain compliance and discipline
- Minimise fat gain when building muscle
- Develop a strong metabolism
- Fine tune results
- Avoid plateaus
- Transform for Life - committment to health being one of the most important factors of your life

You can learn everything you need tracking with The Blueprint in 8 weeks. After this you can return to more intuitive or estimating behaviours.

You will not need to track calories, activity and macronutrients forever.

Starting calories

Note: *If you track using MyFitnessPal you can use the algorithms they present when setting up an account. Guidelines on using MyFitnessPal are available for free on our website* **teambodyproject.com/additional-resources.** *If you don't want to track calories, read about alternative methods in our Tracking chapter.*

Calculating your starting calories - Transform for Life method

IMPORTANT: *If you weigh more than 200 lb (90 kg) use '200 lb' for your calculations*
Note: *2.2 lb = 1 kg*

Multiply bodyweight in pounds by:
- 11.5 for starting weight loss calories
- 13 for starting maintenance
- 15 for starting weight gain

- Multiply the calories x 1.2 if you are male
- Add 150 calories if you are an ectomorph*
- Add 75 calories if you are an ecto-mesomorph*
- Leave calories unchanged if you are a mesomorph*
- Deduct 75 calories if you are an endo-mesomorph*
- Deduct 150 calories if you are an endomorph*
- Deduct 100 kcal per day if you are over 30
- Deduct 150 kcal per day if you are over 40
- Deduct 200 kcal per day if you are over 50

* See pages 231-233 to decide on your body type

Examples

1. Female 160 lb (endomorph) age 45 Goal: Weight loss

160 lb x 11.5 = 1,840 kcal
Endomorph = deduct 150 kcal
Age 45 = deduct 150 kcal
Starting weight loss calories = 1,540 rounded up to 1,550 kcal

2. Male 190 lb (ectomorph). Age 57 Goal: Weight loss

190 lb x 11.5 = 1,840 kcal
Male x 1.2 = 2,208
Ectomorph = add 150 kcal
Age 57 = deduct 200 kcal
Starting weight loss calories = 2,158 rounded down to 2,150 kcal

1. Do not get caught up in how accurate your calories are or hitting them exactly every day.

2. We don't calculate activity into the equation at this stage as it would just be guess work. Be confident in this number as a starting point, knowing it will soon be changed if it is not accurate.

Calorie deficit rules:

- NEVER drop below 1,200 kcal per day.
- Only drop below 1,500 kcal per day if you have the data OR you weigh less than 132 lb (60 kg).
- Never drop calories by more than 500 kcal per day from baseline, regardless of weight.

TASK 4: STARTING CALORIES

Add your starting calories to Your *Health Blueprint* (page 199) or Your *Health Blueprint Light* (page 200).

If you choose not to have a calorie target, write N/A next to *Daily calories.*

LIGHT

Awareness of intake

You do not need to have a calorie target in the first week of your *Blueprint*; or any week.

A large amount of the benefit of tracking intake is based on increased awareness rather than precision of consumption. Therefore, not setting a calorie target and just tracking what you are eating is an excellent starting point and often enough to see considerable results for a long time.

Awareness of how many calories are in certain foods, how many calories are in portions and foods that make you full versus foods that make you hungry is a priceless experience that will support you in the long-term.

A note on tracking calories

When you start tracking calories you will find some foods have more calories in them than you expected and some have less. This can make meeting your calories targets very challenging in the first couple of weeks.

If any of the guidelines suggest (example) 2000 kcal and you are struggling to meet this target, do not try and hit 2000 kcal as a target.

If you are full and you can't eat any more, simply stop eating. Struggling to meet higher calorie targets is particularly likely to be the case if you have introduced higher levels of protein to your diet.

On the other hand, if the guidelines suggest 1500 kcal and you feel too exhausted to work, live and train, do not try and hit 1500 kcal as a target.

If you are not functioning well on lower calories, eat a little more and relax.

The main goal of the first couple of weeks is to gather data, get used to tracking and understand cause and effect, NOT to make you feel uncomfortable.

Note: *Struggling to meet higher calorie targets is particularly likely to be the case if you have introduced higher levels of protein to your diet.*

Lily's Laws

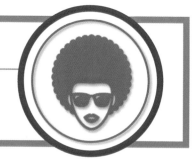

- Calorie balance

Well done. You have taken care of a law of change.

HEALTHY EATING RATIOS

If you want to achieve long-term results, you should focus on sustainable and enjoyable eating from the start. There are a few key aspects of your nutrition we are going to focus on to create your healthy eating *Blueprint*.

1.   Taking into account your likes and dislikes.
2.   Deciding on your healthy/unhealthy ratios.
3.   Compliance as the key metric.

Likes and dislikes

1. **Make a list of 'unhealthy' foods/alcohol you could drop long-term**
Things like soda and fizzy drinks, processed junk foods and microwave meals are common choices.

2. **Make a list of 'unhealthy' foods/alcohol you can't live without**
Some people love a glass of wine, others an ice cream in the park. There is no point in us removing these from your diet if you are going to reintroduce them. We can reduce their intake but removing them entirely creates risk of rebound.

3. **Make a list of 'healthy' foods you enjoy**
What are healthy foods you really enjoy? Check our shopping lists in *Additional Resources: Healthy Nutrition Handbook* to pick out items that really appeal to you.

4. **Make a list of 'healthy' foods you do not enjoy**
Just because broccoli is a so-called 'superfood', if you don't like it don't eat it. There are other vegetables that have a very similar nutrient content.

Note: *We want you to enjoy a long-term sustainable nutrition plan. Sugary, junk type foods and alcohol are NOT an important part of a nutrition plan* **physiologically** *but for some people they are very important* **psychologically**. *By removing them completely, you run the risk of 'rebound' eating after your 'diet' is over.*

Understanding healthy eating ratios

First, we must define what we mean by 'healthy' and 'unhealthy' alongside what healthy means for you.

Healthy:

- Micronutrient (vitamins and minerals) dense
- High fibre
- Satiating (makes you feel full)
- Unprocessed

Healthy for you:

- Within your calorie limits (set in the previous chapter)
- In line with your macronutrient ratios (set later on in *The Blueprint*)

Unhealthy:

- High sugar content
- Processed
- Low micronutrient density
- Not satiating

Unhealthy for you:

- Outside your calorie limits
- Outside your macronutrient ratios

What is generally healthy is going to have a greater impact on all other aspects of your health.

What is healthy *for you* is going to have the greater impact on your body composition and weight.

Deciding on healthy eating ratios

If you want to make progress with your health, you want your ratio to be more healthy than if you are maintaining. A healthy eating ratio is the amount of meals and snacks that are healthy versus the amount of meals and snacks that are unhealthy.

Your choice should be based on consideration of goals, personal preferences and personal compliance capability.

Healthy eating 100% of the time
One of the biggest reasons we have a yo-yo dieting epidemic. The follower of this diet will last one week, three weeks or even 20 weeks. Once they 'break' and eat the forbidden fruit, the floodgates open. We suggest avoiding this at all costs.

Choose this: If you want 'rebound weight' gain.

Healthy/unhealthy eating ratio 95% to 5%
If you are keen on fast results and do better when focused we suggest this ratio. You will be able to fast progress but must still give some consideration to the long-term reality of eating. Try not to neglect the 5%. You should relax on your healthy eating guidelines every 20 meals and every 20 snacks.

Choose this: If you want faster results and have high discipline.

Healthy/unhealthy eating ratio 90% to 10%
This would be ideal for those looking for faster progress. You can relax on your eating guidelines every 10 meals and every 10 snacks.

Choose this: If you want a good level of results.

Healthy/unhealthy eating ratio 80% to 20%
We would still expect some good progress with this ratio. You can relax on your eating guidelines once every five meals and every five snacks.

Choose this: If you are patient for results and find a more balanced approach easier.

Healthy/unhealthy eating ratio 70% to 30%
We would expect maintenance from this ratio. The majority of your meals are healthy, but one meal or snack every day falls outside of guidelines.

Choose this: If you are happy where you are and want to maintain.

Healthy/unhealthy eating ratio less than 70%
If you want to be healthy, the majority of your decisions should be good ones. That is the case for all of us. Once you drop below 70% each further % of drop moves you further from that majority.

Choose this: If you are not committed to a lifetime of health.

TASK 5: HEALTHY EATING RATIOS

Decide on a healthy eating ratio and add to Your *Health Blueprint* (page 199).

LIGHT

Take note of how many foods you eat that are 'healthy' and how many 'unhealthy' when you review the foods you have eaten in the week.
Less than 70% may be harming your goals.

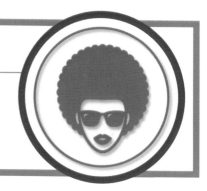

Lily's Laws

- Eat plenty of vegetables
- Limit processed food intake

Well done. You have taken care of TWO laws of change.

'Holiday' ratios

Balance is a pendulum that swings both ways.

If you spend the Christmas holiday eating healthy just 10% of the time, you'll need to spend at least as much time swinging the pendulum the other way. Take charge and make the choice. If you decide you want to spend the two weeks away on holiday eating and drinking merrily, also take the choice that the day you come back you will resume your health and fitness routine.

The secret is not being 'perfect'.

It comes down to having good compliance. You decide how often and for how long you let your hair down.

Implementing healthy eating ratios

Track healthy eating compliance ratios using The Food Compliance Tracker (page 255) located in *Additional Resources*.

FLUX

Many people hit long-term plateaus, rebound weight gain, fail to retain and build muscle, damage metabolism and hit problems with permanent residence in a caloric deficit. You can avoid any of these issues by managing a calorie flux. While a calorie flux may slow down your short-term results a little, you will experience:

- Higher percentage of fat loss
- Fewer plateaus
- Stronger metabolism
- Muscle retention and muscle gain
- Reduced chance of rebound eating

If serious muscle growth and body sculpting is your goal higher calorie weeks are a better option. If muscle retention and maximum fat loss is your goal higher calorie days are a better option.

These are not absolute rules - try different options to see what works best for you.

The following table illustrates how you set out your ratios and flux.

Fat loss flux table

If you have more than 50 lb (23 kg) of weight/fat to lose

Weekly: You can spend 10 weeks in a calorie deficit versus 1 week in a calorie balance.

And/Or

Daily: You can spend 13 days in a calorie deficit for every day in a calorie balance.

If you have between 25 lb (11 kg) and 50 lb of weight/fat to lose

Weekly: You can spend 8 weeks in a calorie deficit versus 1 week in a calorie balance.

And/Or

Daily: You can spend 6 days in a calorie deficit for every day in a calorie balance.

If you have between 10 lb (4.5 kg) and 25 lb of weight/fat to lose

Weekly: You can spend 6 weeks in a calorie deficit versus 1 week in a calorie balance.

And/Or

Daily: You can spend 5 days in a calorie deficit for every 2 days in a calorie balance.

Less than 10lbs to lose

Weekly: You can spend 4 weeks in a calorie deficit versus 1 week in a calorie balance.

And/Or

Daily: You can spend 5 days in a calorie deficit for every 2 days in a calorie balance.

Note 1: You can do both daily and weekly flux but it is not necessary

Note 2: On daily flux, it does not matter if flux days are consecutive

Note 3: You do not need to worry about daily flux on flux weeks.

Increase muscle + reduce fat + retain weight

Weekly: A ratio of one week in surplus versus one week in deficit with a recommended minimum of four weeks in each state.

Note: If you find you are struggling to build muscle, you may need to spend more time in a surplus than in a deficit. This will be a common experience for females, where even a quarter of a pound of additional muscle per week can be a decent return.

AND

Daily: We recommend 1-2 days of flux in both surplus and deficits.
    A.   Higher calorie days when you have heavy training sessions in overall deficit weeks.
    B.   Lower calories on rest days in overall surplus weeks.

Increase muscle mass

Weekly: Up to 8 weeks in surplus versus 1 week in calorie deficit

AND

Daily: We recommend 1 day of lower calorie flux in surplus weeks.
    A.   Lower calories on 1 rest day in overall surplus weeks
    B.   No flux on deficit weeks.

Muscle gain targets should be conservative. Even ¼ lb of muscle in a week is a success. For females ¼ of muscle should be seen as excellent.

Flux is a simple process with three purposes.

1. Protecting your metabolism
2. Providing your body with an opportunity to build muscle
3. Stopping you entering a plateau

How to manage flux

Higher calorie days

1. Increase your calories to bring total calories to 'balance' on 'higher' calorie days. Increase carbs, not protein or fat.

2. Have your higher calorie days on your most intense workout days of the week. NEVER increase calories on rest days.

Note: If muscle growth is your overall goal, higher calorie weeks are usually more effective.

Higher calorie weeks

1. On your higher calorie weeks, increase your calories to 'balance' or above. Increase carbs, not protein or fat.

2. Increase your training intensity and duration on weeks you increase your calorie intake. Resistance should form a higher percentage of your workouts on higher calorie weeks.

Flux calculations

As with all calculations in Transform for Life, there is no absolute rule.

These calculations may be accurate or they may need considerable tweaking to work for you.

Flux calculations based on weight loss calories.

Weight loss kcal	1500 kcal
Balance kcal x 1.3	1950 kcal
Muscle gain kcal x 1.5 kcal	2250 kcal

Calculations with adding/subtracting calories*

Weight loss kcal	1500 kcal
Balance + 500 kcal	2000 kcal
Muscle gain + 750 kcal	2250 kcal

*Simple calorie changes may not as accurate as calculations since adding and subtracting is the same regardless of baseline kcal. However, since none of the calculation can be 100% accurate and will develop based on feedback, I do not find this to be particularly relevant.

Why is the calorie surplus for building muscle usually not as high as for a deficit?

It is harder to build muscle than it is to burn fat. Whilst it is feasible that you can lose 1 lb + of fat week in week out, it is not feasible to build muscle at the same speed.

Note: It is possible, especially in the early stages, to build 1 lb of muscle in a week, so don't worry too much if the scales go up by 1 lb. It may all be muscle.

- If you have **more than 10 lbs** of fat to lose, the surplus for building muscle should be smaller than the deficit for losing fat.
- If you have **less than 10 lbs** of fat lose, the deficit to surplus ratio will be closer to 1/1, although this will be based on:

A.   How quickly you are able to build muscle
B.   How quickly you are able to lose fat

Examples

Woman A struggles to build more than ¼ pound of muscle per week regardless of calorie quantity.
Woman A is able to still lose ½ pound of fat per week in a deficit.
Suitable ratio may be **1 to 2** fat burning/deficit to muscle building/surplus.

AND

Calorie deficits should be slightly higher than calorie surpluses

Man A can comfortably build ½ to 1 pound of muscle per week in a surplus.
Man A struggles to lose more than ½ pound of fat per week in a deficit.
Suitable ratio may be **3 to 2** fat burning/deficit to muscle building/surplus.

AND

Calorie deficits should be slightly lower than calorie surpluses

Woman B can build around ½ pound of muscle per week in a surplus.
Woman B can lose ½ pound of fat per week in a deficit.
Suitable ratio may be **1 to 1** fat burning/deficit to muscle building/surplus

AND

Calorie deficits should be similar to calorie surpluses

Important

Building muscle is a slow process that can't be rushed. Creating small calorie surpluses alongside resistance training is the best way to gain muscle without gaining fat.

Losing the last 10 lbs of fat is a slow process that can't be rushed. (the last 5 lbs can be a very tedious and long process.)

Creating small calorie deficits alongside resistance and cardio training is the best way to lose fat without losing muscle when you already have low body fat.

Flux examples

- **Weight loss daily calories** = 1,700
- **Flux day 'balance' calculation** = 1,700 x 1.3
- **Flux day 'balance' calories** = 2,210
- **Flux daily muscle gain calculation** = 1,700 x 1.45
- **Flux day muscle gain calories** = 2,465

TASK 6: FLUX

Decide on daily and weekly calorie flux and add to Your *Health Blueprint* (page 199).

LIGHT

If you are choosing the *Light* options you will not need to set your ratios and flux, just try and eat more calories on days when you are training and less calories on days when you are not.

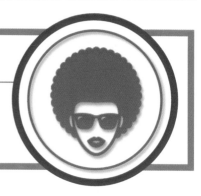

Lily's Laws

- Anabolic and catabolic flux

Well done. You have taken care of a law of change.

MACRONUTRIENT RATIOS

Macronutrient ratios are not a one-size-fits-all solution. There is no way of truly knowing what ratio suits you the best without some trial and error.

Important: *Tracking macronutrients can be overwhelming when you start. Unless you have prior experience with tracking or have been struggling to lose weight for some time, it may be sensible to leave tracking macronutrients until you are comfortable with calories OR you have hit a plateau.*

A macronutrient starting point can be determined based on:

- Body type (outlined on the following pages)
- Goals (performance = higher carbs, fat loss = lower carbs)
- Personal preference

Before setting your starting macronutrient remember the fixed minimums.

- Protein – 30%*
- Carbs – 25%
- Fats – 25%

That gives you just 20% to adjust to taste and goals.

*Vegans and vegetarians usually struggle to meet 30% without supplementation. In this instance, put additional focus on protein availability by eating protein with all meals and snacks.

Body type*

Read the descriptions on the following pages and decide which one best fits your own body type. Be objective. If you aren't sure ask somebody who knows you. This is NOT about how much you currently weigh. An ectomorph can carry lots of excess fat; that does not mean the ectomorph has become an endomorph.

Note: *You can sit between body types. Endo-meso would be a combination of both endomorphic and mesomorphic traits. Ecto-meso would be a combination of both ectomorphic and mesomorphic traits.*

There is some fair contention around the relevance of body types. In my practical experience I have found them useful in guiding starting positions for calories and macronutrients. However, they are by no means absolute and they are certainly not indicative of your ultimate outcome. They are used here for guideline purposes only.

Endomorphs

Endomorphs have a larger bone structure and shorter limbs.

Additional calories consumed do not result in an additional 'need' to burn off calories, making weight gain common.

They are naturally less active and tend to have slower metabolisms. An endomorph would rarely define themselves as 'sporty', and activity and exercise is something they usually have to 'learn' to love.

- Usually shorter than average
- Wider hips and shoulders
- Store fat everywhere

As a rule of thumb, endomorphs do better with lower carbohydrate diets as they have a propensity to insulin response and carb adaptation, making fat loss harder.

Macronutrient starting point: 25% carbs, 40% protein, 35% fat

Mesomorphs

Mesomorphs have a medium bone structure and an athletic overall shape with a natural propensity to build muscle.

They naturally excel at, and enjoy, sports and are normally 'all rounders'.

While mesomorphs have a more natural propensity to build muscle and be lean, they can also gain excess weight if they are inactive and over time become more typical of endomorphs.

- Can be any height
- Wider shoulders with narrow hips
- Store fat on torso and upper limbs (female on glutes and upper thighs too)

As a rule of thumb, as they usually have an effective 'built in' structure for utilizing macronutrients effectively they can function well on most ratios provided calories are correct, so a balanced ratio works best.

Mesomorph Macronutrient starting point: 40% carbs, 30% protein, 30% fat

Endo-mesomorph starting point: 30% carbs, 35% protein, 35% fat

---

Ectomorphs

Ectomorphs have a smaller bone structure and longer limbs. They are typically high energy, fidgeters and any excess calories will be burned off through additional use. The increased 'speed' of an ectomorph's metabolism is less to do with BMR and more to do with NEAT (refer to *The Science* section to learn more about NEAT).

For this reason, they don't do as well with low carb diets, since they tend to use any additional nutrients they consume with extra activity without planning it.

- Usually taller
- Narrower hips and shoulders
- Usually store fat around middle

Macronutrient starting point: 50% carbs, 30% protein, 20% fat

Ecto-mesomorph starting point: 45% carbs, 30% protein, 25% fat

Don't worry about getting your ratio perfect at the start. You will adapt as you go.

TASK 7: MACRONUTRIENT RATIOS

Add your chosen macronutrient ratios to Your *Health Blueprint* (page 199).

LIGHT

Try and eat sufficient carbohydrates, fats and proteins. If any macronutrient is too low, eat a little more of it.

A note on tracking Macronutrients

When you first track macronutrients you will find it almost impossible to meet the targets you have set yourself.

This is not a problem, it is wonderful. Learning about the macronutrient quantities in foods is part of the education. It is one of the most important elements of tracking. Hitting your targeted macronutrients consistently will take you weeks to get right and understand. Don't worry if you struggle to eat enough protein or if your carbohydrates are too high. Trial and error will get you there eventually.

You may find trying to eat 40% protein doesn't work for you and instead choose to focus on small amounts of quality protein in every meal. Alternatively, you may find a protein shake is needed to to make it work.

Enjoy learning about the macronutrient qualities of foods and how you can change them to suit your lifestyle, preferences and goals.

If you have to change your macronutrients because you find it too hard to meet them or it just doesn't fit your lifestyle, relax. It isn't the end of the world and it certainly isn't the end of your *Blueprint*.

Most people make compromises to their initial plans and every moment you spend learning about food, it's macronutrient breakdown and the impact it has on your body is a positive one.

Calorie control, regular exercise and good healthy food ratios are more important for your results than a 10% +/- in carbohydrates/protein.

Lily's Laws

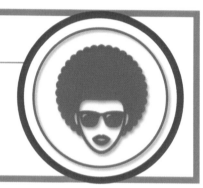

- Sufficient carbohydrates
- Sufficient protein
- Sufficient fat

Well done. You have taken care of THREE laws of change.

Congratulations

Lily's Laws

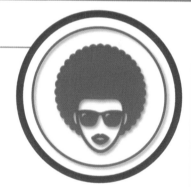

Well done. You've dealt with all of Lily's Laws of Change.

Exercise
- Exercise to stimulate muscle growth and fat loss
- NEAT

Nutrition
- Calorie balance
- Anabolic and catabolic flux
- Sufficient carbohydrates
- Sufficient protein
- Sufficient fat
- Drink enough water
- Eat plenty of vegetables
- Limit processed food intake

Additional nutrition support

To learn more about nutrition, including clearing cupboards and healthy shopping lists, read *The Nutrition* guide, available in *Additional Resources*.

INTRODUCTION TO TRACKING

Tracking is the process of monitoring foods and drinks consumed against movement. It is our proven and recommended method for creating a *Health Blueprint* for life.

I want to make this next point crystal clear.

The best long-term healthy eating system is intuitive eating and NOT tracking.

Intuitive eating, covered below and in *Maintenance Fundamentals* (later in this section) is the ideal end goal for the majority of people. The problem with intuitive eating is that most of us have been attempting to do it our whole lives, and we're not that good at it! We can learn to be good at it – and tracking supports this process.

Tracking is a learning process that helps you discover the foods you respond well to, how many calories and macronutrients are in them, and raises awareness around hunger, appetite, emotional eating and, crucially for results, cause and effect.

Problems with tracking

Before we look at implementing any method, it's important to understand the problems associated with it.

Tracking is the most effective method I have found for building awareness around food intake and achieving sustainable and predictable results, but it is not without its issues.

If any of the below are deal breakers for you, you can choose one of our other methods to support you in pursuit of your goals.

1.   It increases the amount of time we think about food and eating

During the process of tracking you will spend more time thinking about food and experiencing food than you ever have before. If you have a difficult relationship with food, this heightened awareness of food intake and hunger could be a challenge.

For some people, a focus on becoming more aware of thoughts around food decisions is a better option than tracking what is eaten.

Tracking exerts external control on our choices, whereas increasing awareness develops internal control over what we do. Intuitive eating would develop stronger internal control.

For the majority of people both awareness and control are important. I find the conscious relationship that food tracking develops is an important step in changing the way we think about what we eat.

2.   It is very time consuming

For the first week or two it can be a pain as you build up recipe lists and learn what's in certain products. However, most of the benefits you get from tracking will be achieved within 8 short weeks.

After 8 weeks you can move on from tracking with a clear understanding of foods and the impact they have on your body along with a deeper clarity around emotional eating and hunger signals. Once these 8 weeks are done you may find tracking takes much less time and wish to continue or you may choose to stop.

The work you put into tracking will pay you back 100 times over. If lifetime health is your aim, the additional effort of tracking to create *Your Health Blueprint* is worth every moment.

3.   It is not entirely accurate

Tracking calories does not provide you with a cast iron guarantee you will get it right – calorie and macronutrient guidelines on foods can be wrong and people are notoriously bad at tracking accurately.

Although on face value it may seem that tracking is a promise of absolute accuracy, it is not. It is centered on adjusting relative values and building a coachable footprint, not on the promise of precise data.

If you estimate a meal to be 500 kcal and it is actually 600 kcal, this does not matter as much as building a consistent value which can be adapted if necessary. Tracking builds a *Blueprint* that helps you understand perceived quantities and their relationship to your body composition and the scale. Whether you are actually eating 1,800 kcal or 2,000 kcal is less important than understanding what this perceived and relative value does to your body and being able to adapt it.

False reporting or underreporting, where calorie-rich foods like butter and oils are ignored or quantities are vastly underestimated, can be a problem and is covered in *The Plan* chapter.

4.   It supports the consumption of 'unhealthy' foods

Some of the opponents of tracking take issue with the fact that it supports the consumption of 'unhealthy' foods.

Again, this is true. Tracking intake does provide more leeway for consumption of less 'healthy' options. Unlike opponents, I see this as a positive thing.

I believe in the power of choice for the individual. Giving people freedom to eat the foods they want in a sensible way, within a framework, is a valuable option.

If you wish to eat 100% healthy foods and this works for you, the need for tracking is lower – but most people want to eat cake and drink beer. Tracking allows us to develop long-term, sensible approaches to our diet.

Potential contraindications of tracking:

History of eating disorders – if you have a history of eating disorders, it is important you speak with a medical professional before you engage in any dietary control method, including tracking.

Anxiety personality types – some anxiety personality types have a tendency to become obsessed around food intake. This personality type is better suited to throwing away the scales and focusing on *tracking behaviour* or *intuitive eating*.

Why tracking?

It doesn't matter if you eat avocados, nuts, seeds, beef, fish or chocolate, if you eat too much of it you will not lose weight or fat.

Tracking has two purposes:

1.   To set a baseline understanding of your metabolism
2.   To understand which changes to implement

Most people don't sustain healthy weight loss for two reasons:

1.   Lack of knowledge of what they are eating and the impact it has on their body.
2.   Chronic exposure to unnecessarily extreme caloric deficits.

The two go hand in hand.

People don't know what they are eating so when they want to lose weight, they take it to extreme levels.

It's very hard to gauge how much 250-500 calories a day less is, so people end up starving themselves so they can be sure they aren't eating too much.

In the process of writing this book, I was forced to look deep into my own coaching career; the time I spent managing my own weight as a boxer, the time helping fighters make weight and the last few years online supporting thousands of people achieve weight goals.

I've connected the lines between:

A.   The early part of my career when I had sporadic results with personal clients.
B.   The 100% success rate I had to achieve when working with boxers (they didn't get paid if they didn't make weight).
C.   The 90+% success rate I had with personal clients in the latter part of my coaching career.
D.   The frustration I feel seeing people putting in the same effort, yet some achieving goals and others not.

Training weight-class athletes forced me to let go of preconceived ideas and attach to facts.

If you have to weigh 165 lb (75 kg) by August 14th or you don't get paid, you make 165 lb (75 kg) by August 14th. A boxer does not have the option to say:

"I don't understand. I can't lose weight."

When you're dealing in absolutes you realize that a metabolism is entirely predictable. No magic avocados, no mystery and more importantly, no *"Why can't I lose weight?"*

If you track food against activity, people lose weight in a predictable, if not linear way from baseline. If you consider macronutrients and other factors, you can control the factors that influence body composition.

It is ridiculous to assume we can ever exact absolute control over every aspect of our body – we are not machines – but with tracking we manage factors we can influence in a positive way.

Bringing this clinical approach to non-professional athletes needs to be accompanied by sustainability and built around lifestyles, but the fundamentals remain.
As a coach, I had a rule:

If you choose not to track what you are eating (including butter, oils, sauces, picking from kids' plates, tasting while cooking and all the other underreported areas), I can't promise results!

I can support you, help you, guide you, and get the most out of your workouts, but I can't coach your weight management.

Unlike with professional athletes, where control is the centerpiece, results come for different reasons:

- People can eat things they love in larger quantities than they had imagined
- People take leaps forwards with emotional eating
- People are surprised by how much they enjoy understanding their body
- People enjoy predictability of outcomes
- People learn that every decision (including the 'couple' of chips they have from their partners' plate) makes a difference – but that sometimes the difference is not big enough to matter!
- People become aware of cause and effect

For predictable and repeatable results, nothing comes close to tracking – and I have tried everything!

It allows for mistakes, balance and eating foods you love, but it needs you to keep track of it.

Other options

If you decide you don't want to track, we have provided guidelines on portion control, intuitive eating and behaviour tracking.

Intuitive eating is important for everybody in the long-term.

Within the context of everything else in the *Transform for Life* guidelines, these alternative methods should still be very effective.

TASK: DECIDE ON A TRACKING OPTION:

Option 1: Macronutrient tracking (pages 186-187)
Option 2: Portion control (pages 188-189)
Option 3: Intuitive eating (pages 189-191)
Option 4: Behaviour tracking (pages 191-192)

Option 1: Macronutrient tracking

The principles of macronutrient tracking are:

- Record all food and drink consumed

Advantages:

- The most accurate method
- Easiest to implement changes and manipulate results
- Leaves a footprint; creating a clear picture of dietary habits over time

Disadvantages:

- Time-consuming in the early stages
- Reporting can be inaccurate – see *Underreporting*

Macronutrient tracking is suitable for people who:

- Want to enjoy foods that are not on a 'healthy' list
- Want to achieve consistent and repeatable results
- Are dedicated to getting the data for long-term change
- Want the most accurate and effective transformation system

Macronutrient tracking is not suitable for people who:

- Have a history of certain eating disorders
- Do not have any time to record data, even in the short-term
- Are happy with weight, fat and muscle levels

Implementing Your Method – Macronutrient and Calorie Tracking

Whether you are following *The Blueprint* or *The Blueprint Light* we strongly recommend you use *MyFitnessPal* to track your calories and macronutrients.

Follow our *MyFitnessPal* guidelines by visiting the following link:

www.teambodyproject.com/additional-resources

TASK

Using our guidelines, set up an account on *myfitnesspal* before you continue creating *Your Health Blueprint*.

You may find the tracking experience a little overwhelming at first and that is both understandable and natural but remember:

1.   The tracking process is not forever. Very, very few people track for longer than 8-12 weeks. It is a system of discovery around the cause and effect of food, not a lifetime habit.

2.   This system has come from a professional sports environment, where accuracy of information was the difference between winning and losing – you don't need this level of precision.

If you find the thought of tracking your food intake, macronutrients and health a little overwhelming, follow this three-step system to ease yourself into the process without any pressure.

Three-step system

1. **Just track it**

    Don't worry about how much you are eating, what you are eating or why you are eating it.

    Just track it!

    This will raise a new-found awareness around food that will start your process of change.

2. **Calorie balance**

    Once you get used to tracking food and activity, you can attempt to create a calorie deficit, if weight loss is important to you. This will be much easier when you understand the calorie quantities of foods.

    You do not have to be perfect. If you are over or under your calories by 10% or so, it doesn't matter.

3. **Track your macronutrients**

    Once you get used to creating a calorie deficit you can start attempting to hit macronutrients.

ALTERNATIVE TRACKING METHODS

Macronutrient tracking is not for everybody. For some it is too time consuming, even in the short-term.

The below methods have proven levels of efficacy and can be used alongside the rest of the guidance within *Transform for Life*.

Option 2: Portion control

With portion control you assess the food on your plate using a variety of methods.

The method we recommend is based on using our hands to judge the amount of foods and make suitable adaptations.

The principles of portion control are:

- Use hands to measure the amount of food eaten

Advantages:

- A simple method of portion control
- Once you understand principles, it is easy to implement
- Time friendly

Disadvantages:

- Harder to make small changes
- Not as accurate as macronutrient tracking
- Doesn't leave a 'footprint' of behaviours to revert back to

Portion control is suitable for people who:

- Want a simple method of managing portions
- Are not as interested in 'fine tuning' results
- Don't have time to record everything

Portion control is not suitable for people who:

- Have very specific goals
- Are already happy with weight, fat and muscle levels
- Want to build up a footprint of changes

Implementing Your Method – Portion Control

The best thing about the portion control method is no measuring devices or calculators are required. All you need is your hands. After all, your hands are with you everywhere you go!

It is true that some people have large or small hands for their size, but it is an easy-to-implement starting point for portion control.

As with every other method, portion control only creates a starting point, after which hunger, weight loss and body changes will dictate how you adapt. For every meal you have, simply calculate your portions based on the 'hand measured' sizes suggested below.

Calculating Macronutrients

How to calculate protein required in each meal
Men: 2 palms of protein
Women: 1-1.5 palms of protein
Protein: Eggs, chicken, turkey, white fish, steak, cottage cheese
A palm-sized portion is roughly the same width and diameter as your palm.

How to calculate vegetables required in each meal
Men: 2 fists of vegetables
Women: 1-1.5 fist of vegetables
Vegetables: Spinach, carrots, kale, watercress, broccoli, etc.
A fist-sized portion is roughly the same width and diameter as your fist.

How to determine carbohydrates required in each meal
Men: 2 cupped hands of carbohydrates
Women: 1-1.5 cupped hands of carbohydrates
Carbs: Grains, potatoes, fruits, etc.
A cupped hand is roughly what you could fit inside your palm.

How to determine fats required in each meal
Men: 2 thumb sizes of fat
Women: 1-1.5 thumb sizes of fat
Fats: Nuts, oils, butters, seeds, etc.

If you use the rough estimates above to set a baseline, you can use our modification guidelines to adapt as you go.

Option 3: Intuitive eating

If you follow the fundamentals of *Transform for Life* alongside intuitive eating, you will almost certainly achieve results in the short-term.

In the medium-term, specific results cannot always be guaranteed with this approach, creating frustration. If we have developed a sound understanding of how our body is responding to foods it can be very effective but for many people this isn't the case and results are slow.

In the long-term, once goals are met, intuitive eating is the best method for the majority of people – although not all.

Note: *The principles of intuitive eating should be implemented by everybody, regardless of tracking method.*

The principles of intuitive eating are:

- Eat slowly
- Stop eating before you feel full
- Focus on fibre rich and voluminous foods
- Ensure high protein, high carbs, high fat and vegetables
- Tune in to hunger signals and separate actual hunger from emotional hunger
- Make peace with food – don't see food as good or bad

Advantages:

- No tracking required
- Easy to implement
- Perfect if general health is the goal, rather than weight loss
- Excellent for long-term maintenance

Disadvantages:

- Hard/impossible to coach and make precise alterations
- Requires a higher quantity of healthy whole foods to work well
- Difficult to implement for somebody coming directly from a lifetime of poor choices

Intuitive eating is suitable for people who:

- Can follow healthier diets without danger of rebound eating
- Cannot bear to track and just want to be healthy
- Have spent a period of time tracking and feel confident in macronutrient and calorie control; nobody should have to track forever unless they want to

Intuitive eating is not suitable for people who:

- Like to build a higher quantity of non-healthy foods into their diet
- Have specific physical appearance goals
- Like data and trackable progress
- Want to find a baseline of information to work from for the future

Implementing Your Method – Intuitive Eating

If you want to rely on Intuitive eating as your chosen method of portion control, it's important you are committed to having a slightly higher ratio of healthy eating.

Processed and refined foods have different impacts on hormones (such as ghrelin, leptin and insulin) than non-refined foods, making it much harder to make decisions mindfully.

To use intuitive eating you must first learn the difference between hunger and appetite:

- Hunger is the need to eat
- Appetite is the desire to eat
- Appetite can be ignored, hunger should not be ignored; if you are to be successful with mindful eating, you must learn to recognize the difference

How to implement:

- Pay close attention to signs of satiety. Satiety is the satisfied feeling of being full after eating
- Eat filling foods. Empty calories leave you hungry for more and disrupt our ability to tune in to food requirements
- Go for nutrient-dense foods that fill you up. High-fibre fruits, vegetables, proteins and whole grains beat hunger pangs and can help you resist temptations

Intuitive eating checklist:

- Put reminders in the cutlery draw and on the table to eat slowly and consciously
- Stop frequently during eating times to check you are still hungry
- Never eat snacks until at least 15 minutes **after** hunger strikes
- Always drink water as the first option when hunger strikes
- Differentiate between hunger and appetite; see *The Art of Change – Emotional eating*

With an understanding of the importance of calorie balance, healthy food ratios, calorie flux, macronutrients and the importance of exercise, intuitive eating could work very well for you.

Intuitive eating will make some of our specific coaching methods harder, but certainly not impossible to implement.

Use our shopping lists in the *Nutrition Handbook* in the *Additional Resources* section to stack your cupboard with the foods that can fit into any healthy meal plan.

You can find our *10 Principles of Intuitive Eating* checklist in the *Trackers* chapter of *Additional Resources*.

Option 4: Behaviour tracking

I love the idea of people throwing away the scales and focusing on doing healthy things or 'tracking behaviours' as the goal.

I wish this concept would find more mainstream appeal, but people want visible results and tracking behaviours does not take calorie balance into account.

The principles of tracking behaviours are:

- Your 'metric' becomes what you do, not what you achieve
- Throw away the scales and measuring tape for good
- Work hard at self acceptance

Advantages:

- No tracking required
- Easy to implement
- Perfect if general health is the goal, rather than weight loss
- Excellent for long-term maintenance

Disadvantages :

- Tangible results cannot be guaranteed
- Most people are more satisfied working towards a concrete goal

Tracking behaviours is suitable for people who:

- Cannot bear to track and just want to be healthy
- Have spent a period of time tracking and feel confident in macronutrient and calorie control; nobody should have to track forever
- Like ticking boxes

Tracking behaviours is not suitable for people who:

- Like to build a higher quantity of non-healthy foods into their diet
- Have specific physical appearance goals
- Like data and trackable progress
- Want to find a baseline of information to work from for the future

Implementing your method - Tracking behaviours

- Eat healthy meals as a goal
- Exercise every day as a goal
- Drink plenty of water as a goal
- Avoid junk foods as a goal
- Walk steps as a goal
- There are no scales or measuring tapes

If this is the way you want to do things, you can't step on the scales every few weeks and hope you've lost a few pounds as that will lead to disappointment and you are better off tracking from the start.

If you let go of tracking and weighing and replace it with a focus on tracking health behaviours, your accountability, goal and result are based on the amount of behaviours you have done rather than the measurements or scales.

Be proud of accomplishing healthy behaviours.

In the *Additional Resources* section there are a few features that will help you track behaviours:

- Food Compliance Tracker
- Exercise Compliance Tracker
- Behaviour Tracker

MEASUREMENTS

If you want to know that what you are doing is working, you'll need to take measurements to check against.

As a general rule of thumb you can take:

- Weight weekly
- Measurements bi-weekly
- A photograph monthly

Weight

We suggest against weighing every day as it can fluctuate with water retention and cause unnecessary concern. We recommend weighing weekly as it gives you the opportunity to 'steer the ship' if the results aren't what you were expecting.

Calibrating scales

Find something heavy that is a fixed weight like a dumbbell (over 7 lb / 3 kg).

- Before you weigh yourself, first weigh an object to ensure the scales have not changed the calibration point
- Check the weight of the object a couple of times
- Recheck the weight of the object every week before you weigh yourself to check calibration

Creating similar conditions before weight is taken

1. Eat your last meal of the day as early as possible on the evening before. Make this the same time you eat your final meal every evening before weighing and measuring.
2. Weigh yourself after any bathroom toilet habits and before any drinks or foods in the morning at the same time.
3. Weigh yourself completely naked or with underwear only.

This time of the week, every week is the only time you weigh yourself – after eating at the same time the night before and following the same protocol in the morning.

TASK 8: MEASUREMENTS

Add your weight and measurements to *Your Health Blueprint* (page 199) or *Your Health Blueprint Light* (page 200).

A note on single measurements

Never take the number on the scales on any given week too seriously and certainly don't panic and make drastic changes one way or another. Whether you've lost 4 lb (1.8 kg) or gained 1 lb (0.45 kg) in a single week is not necessarily indicative of your overall direction. If you consistently don't lose weight or consistently gain weight, that is when you should respond.

Taking measurements

You should take your measurements every two weeks and if you're going to do it, you should have a decent measuring tape that you can use easily. Take measurements after you have weighed yourself. Always tighten the tape to a snug fit.

Shoulder:	Measure at the widest point of the shoulders. Measure after a normal rather than forced exhalation.
Chest:	Measure across the nipple line. Measure after a normal rather than forced exhalation.
Upper arm:	Measure at the halfway point between elbow and top of shoulder with an unflexed arm. Measure to this point if you have to.
Waist:	Measure across the belly button. Relax and measure after a normal exhalation.
Hips:	Measure at the widest point.
Thigh:	Measure halfway between the knee and the thigh crease.

TASK

Add measurements to *Your Health Blueprint* or *Your Health Blueprint Light*.

Taking a photograph

Take a full body photograph:

- Directly front on
- Directly back to camera
- Facing to one side

Take all future photographs in the same room under the same lighting conditions. If you retake your photos every month you should see a significant difference in your image and it is a very visual way of tracking your progress over a period of time.

GETTING EQUIPPED

For workouts:

- Dumbbells (see *Buying the correct weights* on the following page)
- Exercise mat
- Water bottle
- Towel
- Comfortable exercise clothes
- Suitable training shoes (for most people 'cross trainers' are the best option for home workouts)

For measuring:

- Calibrated scales
- Measuring tape

For nutrition:

- Containers for prepared food
- A good blender or juicer
- Protein shaker for shakes and smoothies
- Non-stick frying pan

Watching workouts via your TV

If you have a modern television, it may have a web browser built in, allowing you to watch workouts directly from the TBP website. If not, you still have a few good options:

From a PC or laptop
PCs and laptops may be connected to a television using either:

- A suitable HDMI cable
- A VGA cable (usually a blue connector)
- A DVI cable

Note: *Neither VGA nor DVI carry audio, so you will need to use your computer's speakers.*

From a MacBook:

- Pre-2017 models require a Mini DisplayPort (Thunderbolt) to HDMI adapter
- 2017-onwards will need a USB3 to HDMI or USB3 to VGA adapter

From an Android phone or tablet:

- You may be able to connect wirelessly to your television if both your Android device and television support DLNA
- A suitable USB to HDMI adapter

From an iPhone or iPad:

- A Lightning to HDMI adapter
- If your television supports AirPlay, you can connect your device wirelessly

Buying the correct weights

Beginner female dumbbell set

Unless you can afford it or already own them, there is little point in purchasing weights that are 1 kg or less. You will soon grow out of them and can use water bottles or other household items instead.

Note: *1 kg = 2.2 lb*

1. **First set (light).** Your starting 'light' weight should be around 2 kg (4-5 lb).
   (**Note:** *if you are using 1 kg for 'light' this will become your medium weight.*)

2. **Second set (medium).** Having a 'medium' weight of around 3-4 kg (6-9 lb) would be hugely beneficial.

3. **Third set (heavy).** After a time, you may feel like exercises such as squat variations are proving too easy with 3-4 kg weights and at this point we would recommend purchasing an additional set of dumbbells of 5-6 kg (10-14 lb).

Beginner male dumbbell set

1. **First set (light).** Your starting 'light' weight should be around 3 kg (6-7 lb).
   (**Note:** *if you are using 1 kg for 'light' this can become your 'medium' weight.*)

2. **Second set (medium).** Having a 'medium' weight of around 4-5 kg (8-12 lb) would be hugely beneficial.

3. **Third set (heavy).** After a time, you will feel like exercises such as squat variations are proving too easy with 4-5 kg weights and at this point we would recommend purchasing an additional set of dumbbells of 7-8 kg (14-20 lb).

Note: *These are rough guidelines only and you should adjust according to your own strength and capabilities.*

FINALISING YOUR BLUEPRINT

Your Health Blueprint: example

1. Fitness test score	16
2. Exercise plan	Apprentice Plan (The Journey)
3. NEAT target	10,000 steps
4. Starting calories	2,150

5. Healthy eating ratios	Healthy eating	Unhealthy eating
	90%	10%

6. Daily Flux ratios/Weekly flux ratios	Daily ratio	Weekly ratio
	5 / 6	2 / 1

7. Macronutrient ratios	Carbs	Fat	Protein
	45%	30%	25%

8. Measurements and weight

Shoulders	58" / 147 cm
Chest	44" / 112 cm
Upper arm	18" / 46 cm
Waist	36" / 91 cm
Hips	33" / 84 cm
Upper leg	24" / 61 cm
Starting weight	185 lb / 84 kg

Additional Blueprints are available to print out by visiting:

www.teambodyproject.com/additional-resources

Your Health Blueprint Light: example

1. Fitness test score	16
2. Exercise plan	Apprentice Plan (The Journey)
3. NEAT target	10,000 steps
4. Starting calories	2,150

8. Measurements and weight

Shoulders	58" / 147 cm
Chest	44" / 112 cm
Upper arm	18" / 46 cm
Waist	36" / 91 cm
Hips	33" / 84 cm
Upper leg	24" / 61 cm
Starting weight	185 lb / 84 kg

You should now be able to complete your chosen *Health Blueprint* confidently using the templates on the following pages. Once your *Blueprint* is complete then you will be ready to start *The Plan*.

Additional *Blueprints* are available to print out by visiting:

www.teambodyproject.com/additional-resources

YOUR HEALTH BLUEPRINT

1. Fitness test score	
2. Exercise plan	
3. NEAT target	
4. Starting calories	

	Healthy eating	Unhealthy eating
5. Healthy eating ratios		

	Daily ratio	Weekly ratio
6. Daily Flux ratios/Weekly flux ratios		

	Carbs	Fat	Protein
7. Macronutrient ratios			

8. Measurements and weight

Shoulders	
Chest	
Upper arm	
Waist	
Hips	
Upper leg	
Starting weight	

YOUR HEALTH BLUEPRINT LIGHT

1. Fitness test score	
2. Exercise plan	
3. NEAT target	
4. Starting calories	

8. Measurements and weight

Shoulders	
Chest	
Upper arm	
Waist	
Hips	
Upper leg	
Starting weight	

AN OBJECTIVE APPROACH

Most 'diets' are focused on maximising results early on to prove the efficacy of the dietary protocol and solidify the validity of the method in the mind of the dieter.

This approach is short term. Any deviation from progress signals failure, and therein lies the potential for total abandonment of the health plan in favour of less favourable habits.

I call this the subjective approach - the entire basis of the method relies on weight loss and/or relevant progress being made.

With *Transform for Life* we see all outcomes as favourable. Every week presents us with fresh data that supports fine tuning our Blueprint until we discover a way of approaching health that works for us; not just for results, but for compliance and enjoyability.

This objective approach allows us to see every week as beneficial, regardless of whether we achieved what we set out to achieve - the knowledge we gather being the valuable asset as we learn to adapt based on outcome. There is no failure with Transform for Life, only learning through trial.

Fine tuning is not just the reserve of improving outcomes either, it is also used to find a sustainable, long term health plan - and that can mean results are compromised in favour of sustainability.

For instance, many people will struggle at first to meet protein targets. Protein levels for maximum fat loss and muscle growth are higher than most people would naturally choose to eat.

The vast majority of professional athletes, bodybuilders and even serious recreational athletes and exercisers will use a supplement to help them reach the 'ideal' protein levels they require for repair and adaptation.

If you have set a target of 40% protein and you struggle to meet 25% within a diet that you find preferable, you have a choice to make based on this newfound knowledge:

A.   Lower your protein targets to be in line with your dietary preferences.
B.   Consider adding a protein shake or bar to your diet to meet your protein targets.
C.   Change your usual dietary preferences (more meat, less grains etc) to support you in meeting your protein targets.

None of these options is right or wrong. It may be considered that option A has the highest chance of long term compliance and C the least.

B and C may allow for more precise results (and for athletes this is the driving force)but option A would not block results for the majority. Provided other factors like calorie balance, healthy ratios and exercise quantities were considered, results would still be outstanding.

Weight loss

On most dietary protocols, failure to lose weight signals an unsuccessful week. At Transform for Life weight gain, weight balance and weight loss are treated as equals within the same overall story - all three being relevant within your life of health.

- A week of weight gain can be observed and implemented when muscle building is your goal.
- A week of weight balance can be observed and implemented when maintenance becomes the goal.
- A week of weight loss can observed and understood as a week that supports fat loss.

Looking objectively, rather than subjectively at our weekly outcome, we can learn and adapt/iterate to ensure the next week we are closer to understanding our own ideal balance.

One swallow doesn't make a summer

This message is so important, we will repeat it regularly.

Let's imagine you eat a daily diet of 1800 kcal this week alongside 5 workouts and 10,000 steps a day.

At the end of the week you weigh exactly the same. Does this mean you need to reduce your calories further to continue making progress?

It may do, but equally it may not. Results are never linear and should be averaged out as much as possible; the more data you have the more confidently you can make a conclusive answer.

Example:

If your weight doesn't change at 1800 kcal (assuming your reporting is accurate) for one week there is not enough data to assume your calorie levels are too high for weight loss.

Suggested adaptation: Leave calories alone.

If you don't lose weight on 1800 kcal (assuming your reporting is accurate) for two weeks, you possibly need to drop calories and/or increase exercise/NEAT.

Suggested adaptation: Drop calories, but keep an eye out for excessive weight loss (more than 2 lbs weight loss per week average).

If you don't lose weight on 1800 kcal (assuming your reporting is accurate) for three weeks, you almost certainly need to drop calories and/or increase exercise/NEAT.

Suggested adaptation: Drop calories, but still keep an eye out for excessive weight loss (more than 2 lbs weight loss per week average).

If you don't lose weight on 1800 kcal (assuming your reporting is accurate) for four weeks, you can confidently say that you need to be at a lower level to make suitable progress.

We must always keep our minds open and objective. Try and approach your health plan the way an objective and invested coach would.

A final point

Approaching health objectively is not possible for everybody.

If you have a history of eating disorders, high anxiety around your physique or generalised emotional attachment to numbers on the scale, we would recommend following a less objective and outcome focused health model.

Tracking behaviours and intuitively eating are far more suitable approaches in these instances. Both of these methods are outlined in this book and both are capable of yielding impressive results.

THE FIRST WEEK

The first week of your journey is going to lay down the benchmark for your long-term results. You should be clear on what you are doing this week based on *Your Health Blueprint*.

Refer back to *Your Health Blueprint* if needed:

1. Follow the workout plan based on your realistic long-term exercise targets created at the beginning of *The Blueprint*. (pages 157-158)
2. Follow a nutrition plan based on the Blueprint Guidelines in *Getting Started with Nutrition*. (pages 161-181)
3. Follow your tracking method selected in the Tracking chapter. (pages 182-191)
4. Check measurements against baseline as set out in Measurements.(pages 193-194)

Don't put too much pressure on yourself to get it right; the most important aspect of week one is not about being perfect but rather tracking what you do.

This data will enable you to make intelligent decisions (raising calories, dropping calories, eating more protein, eating less carbs, doing more exercise, doing less exercise, being more active, changing flux ratios, changing healthy eating ratios) over the coming weeks and months.

You do not have to track forever.

Beyond tracking, try and keep a note of soft metrics:

- Hunger levels
- Cravings
- Energy levels
- Emotions
- Sleep quality
- Hydration
- Enjoyment of workouts

You'll find a Soft Metrics Tracker chart (pages 256-257) in *Additional Resources*.

Once you are confident with what you are going to do next week and how you are going to measure it... you're ready to *Transform for Life!*

ANALYSIS OF OUTCOMES

At the end of week one, you should retake your weight and measurements under the same conditions as the previous week. While we normally recommend measurements every two weeks, for this first week you should measure and weigh. Once your measurements and body weight are taken, you can compare your results to the charts below and note the relevant **letter and number.**

Note: *There is separate guidance in each table for tracking, portion control and intuitive eating. Choose depending on which method you follow.*

Bodyweight (note which letter best represents your outcome)

A.	Gained more than > 1 kg or 2 lb* (pages 205-206)
B.	Gained between 0-1 kg or 2 lb (Pages 206-208)
C.	No change (pages 209-211)
D.	Lost between 0-1 kg or 2 lb (pages 211-212)
E.	Lost more than < 1 kg or 2 lb**(pages 213-214)

---

* If your weight gain is more than 2 lb (0.9 kg) in a single week do not worry. Change your plan according to the guidelines recommended in coaching table A.

** If you have had a result that is significantly more than 2 lbs weight loss, change your data according to the following rules in coaching table E.

Very important caveat:
- If you have less than 10 lbs of weight to lose, you should not aim to lose more than 1 lb of weight in any given week. If you lose more than 1 lb adjust according to E)
- If you have less than 5 lbs of weight to lose, you should not aim to lose more than 1/2 lbs of weight in any given week. If you lose more than 1/2 lb adjust according to E)

For the majority, between 1- 2 lbs of weight will be fine, but for those with lower body fat this indicates a potential for muscle loss - the coaching tables need adjusting accordingly.

Measurements (note which number best represents your outcome)

1.	Gained measurements in ALL areas
2.	Gained measurements in some areas and stayed the same in others
3.	Gained measurements in some areas and lost in other areas
4.	No change
5.	Lost measurements in some areas and stayed the same in others
6.	Lost measurements in ALL areas

Read the following BEFORE making changes to your nutrition and exercise plan.

1. Avoid panic changes: In the first week you may see dramatic changes, such as 5 lb (2.2 kg) or more weight loss, unexpected weight gain and/or dramatic measurement changes up or down. You have made some profound changes that could impact your levels of water retention significantly in either direction so it is important not to overreact to any single event.

2. You don't have to make changes every week just because you stop losing weight. It is likely you will lose weight one week, stabilize the next, and so on. The following guidelines would be applied to patterns seen over two or more weeks (with the exception of the first week when adjustments are made regardless).

Using the coaching tables

The following tables are broad coaching guidelines for dynamically adapting your plan based on a desire for fat loss and muscle retention as a primary goal.

Weight change A) with measurement outcome 1 – 4

> **Nutrition action plan**
>
> **Tracking:** Your calorie levels are too high for fat loss and too high for optimal muscle building. Reduce calories by **up to** 500 kcal per day.
>
> **Portion control:** Make balanced but noticeable reductions to all of your portion sizes.
>
> **Intuitive eating:** Stop eating earlier than you think you should. Consider removing one snack per day from your diet.

and

> **Exercise action plan**
>
> I. If you are working out for less than 450 minutes TOTAL per week consider adding a cardio workout or sculptor up to twice a week either AFTER your current workout OR on alternative days.
>
> II. Increase NEAT (steps and general non-exercise movement).
>
> **Note:** *Effective exercise range is between 150 and 450 minutes per week.*

Weight change A) with measurement outcome 5 – 6

Nutrition action plan

Tracking: Your calorie levels are too high for fat loss and too high for optimal muscle building. Reduce calories by up to 500 kcal per day.

Portion control: Make balanced but noticeable reductions to all of your portion sizes.

Intuitive eating: Stop eating before you think you should. Consider removing one snack per day from your diet.

Note: *While you have improved your measurements, gaining more than 2.2 lb (1 kg) per week in MUSCLE is not sustainable and you will start increasing fat levels at your current caloric intake.*

and

Exercise action plan

I.   If you are working out for less than 450 minutes TOTAL per week consider adding a cardio workout up to twice a week if you have time, either AFTER your current workout OR on alternative days.

II.   Increase NEAT (steps and general non-exercise movement).

Note: *Effective exercise range is between 150 and 450 minutes per week.*

The overall focus for an **A)** body weight change is reducing calories AND increasing expenditure. Because your weight gain was more than 2 lb (0.9 kg), consider making changes in both nutrition and exercise.

If your weight change was in group **B)** use the following tables to help you make changes for the next week.

Weight change B) with measurement outcome 1 – 2

Nutrition action plan

Tracking: Reduce calories by up to 250 kcal per day. Predominantly reduce your carbohydrate quantity unless carbohydrates are already less than 25%.

Portion control: Reduce the size of the portions in the majority of your meals.

Intuitive eating: Stop eating before you feel full. Consider removing a snack on most days.

OR

Exercise action plan

I.   If you are working out for less than 450 minutes TOTAL per week, consider adding a cardio workout, either AFTER your current workout OR on alternative days.

II.   Increase NEAT (steps and general non-exercise movement).

Note: Effective exercise range is between 150 and 450 minutes per week.

Weight change B) with measurement outcome 3 – 4

Nutrition action plan

Tracking: Your calorie levels are too high for fat loss. Reduce calories by up to 250 kcal per day.

Portion control: Reduce the size of the portions in the majority of your meals.

Intuitive eating: Stop eating before you feel full. Consider removing a snack on most days.

OR

Exercise action plan

I.   If you are working out for less than 450 minutes TOTAL per week, consider adding a cardio workout, either AFTER your current workout OR on alternative days.

II.   Increase NEAT (steps and general non-exercise movement).

Note: Effective exercise range is between 150 and 450 minutes per week.

Weight change B) with measurement outcome 5 – 6

Nutrition action plan

Tracking: Reduce calories by up to 250 kcal per day. Your calorie levels are too high for weight loss but your macronutrient balance and exercise quantity is excellent for muscle building. This week represents an ideal balance for building muscle without gaining fat. *

Portion control: Reduce the size of the portions in the majority of your meals.

Intuitive eating: Stop eating before you feel full. Consider removing a snack on most days.

*Provided your weight gain is not more than 1/2 lb for females and 1 lb for males. If weight gain is more than 1 lb this may represent muscle **and** fat gain. Ideal muscle gain is 0.5 - 1 lb for males and 0.25 to 0.5 lbs for females.

OR

Exercise action plan

I.   If you are working out for less than 450 minutes TOTAL per week, consider adding a cardio workout, either AFTER your current workout OR on alternative days.

II.   Increase NEAT (steps and general non-exercise movement).

Note: *Effective exercise range is between 150 and 450 minutes per week.*

The overall focus of change for a **B)** body weight change is reducing calories OR increasing expenditure. If your weight gain was more than 1 lb (0.45 kg), consider making changes in either nutrition or exercise. You can make changes in both, but it may not be necessary.

If your weight change was in group **C)** use the following tables to help you make changes for the next week.

Weight change C) with measurement outcome 1 – 2

Nutrition action plan

Tracking: Your calorie levels are too high for fat loss and your carb quantity may be too high. Reduce calories by up to 250 kcal per day.

Portion control: Reduce the size of the portions in the majority of your meals. Your calorie levels are too high for weight loss and your carb levels may be too high. The majority of your portion reduction should be from carbohydrates unless carbohydrates are already low.

Intuitive eating: Your calorie levels are too high for fat loss. Consider reducing the amount of carb-based foods you eat unless your carbs are already low.

Note: Never reduce carbohydrates if they are already less than approximately 25% of your diet.

OR

Exercise action plan

I.   If you are working out for less than 450 minutes TOTAL per week consider adding a cardio workout either AFTER your current workout OR on alternative days.

II.   Increase NEAT (steps and general non-exercise movement).

Note: Effective exercise commitment is between 150 and 450 minutes per week.

Weight change C) with measurement outcome 3 – 4

Nutrition action plan

Tracking: Your calorie levels are too high for fat loss. Reduce calories by up to 250 kcal per day with the the majority of the reduction coming from carbohydrates, especially on non-training days.

Portion control: Your calorie levels are too high for fat loss. Reduce carbs in some meals, especially on non-training days.

Intuitive eating: Your calorie levels are too high for fat loss. Eat less carbs, especially on days when you are not training.

Note: *Never reduce carbohydrates if they are already less than approximately 25% of your diet.*

OR

Exercise action plan

I.   If you are working out for less than 450 minutes TOTAL per week consider adding a resistance or cardio workout either AFTER your current workout OR on alternative days.

II.   Increase NEAT (steps and general non-exercise movement).

Note: *Effective exercise commitment is between 150 and 450 minutes per week.*

Weight change C) with measurement outcome 5 – 6

Nutrition action plan

Tracking: Reduce calories by up to 250 kcal per day to lose fat and weight . Your calorie levels are too high for weight loss but this week represents an excellent long-term balance.

Portion control: Your calorie levels are too high for fat loss. Reduce carbs in some meals, especially on non-training days.

Intuitive eating: Your calorie levels are too high for fat loss. Eat less carbs, especially on days when you are not training.

Note: *This week represents an excellent long-term balance based on your current situation.*

OR

Exercise action plan

I. If you are working out for less than 450 minutes TOTAL per week consider adding a resistance or cardio workout either AFTER your current workout OR on alternative days.

II. Increase NEAT (steps and general non-exercise movement).

Note: Effective exercise commitment is between 150 and 450 minutes per week.

The overall focus for a **C)** weight change is reducing calories or considering your macronutrient balance. Because your weight hasn't changed, consider making adjustments in either nutrition or exercise. Making changes in both would not be necessary to make progress.

If your weight change was in group **D)** use the following tables to help you make changes for the next week.

Weight change D) with measurement outcome 1 – 2*

Nutrition action plan

Tracking: Your calorie levels are ideal for weight loss but your macronutrient balance may be off for fat loss. Consider increasing your protein levels and/or decreasing your quantity of carbohydrates.**

Portion control: Your calorie levels are ideal for weight loss but your macronutrient balance may be off for fat loss. Consider increasing your protein levels and/or decreasing your quantity of carbohydrates.**

Intuitive eating: Your calorie levels are ideal for weight loss but your macronutrient balance may be off for fat loss. Consider increasing your protein levels and/or decreasing your quantity of carbohydrates.**

*Please consider water retention as a possibility.
**Don't reduce carbs lower than 25% of total. Don't increase protein levels to higher than 50% of total.

OR

Exercise action plan

If you are working out for less than 450 minutes TOTAL per week consider adding a Sculptor workout AFTER your current workout.

Note: Effective exercise commitment is between 150 and 450 minutes per week.

Weight change D) with measurement outcome 3 – 4

Nutrition action plan

Tracking: Your calorie levels are ideal for weight loss but your macronutrient balance may be off for fat loss.**

Portion control: Your calorie levels are ideal for weight loss but your macronutrient balance may be off for fat loss. Consider increasing your protein levels and/or decreasing your quantity of carbohydrates.**

Intuitive eating: Your calorie levels are ideal for weight loss but your macronutrient balance may be off for fat loss. Consider increasing your protein levels and/or decreasing your quantity of carbohydrates.**

**Do not reduce carbs lower than 25% of total. Do not increase protein levels to higher than 50% of total.

Exercise action plan

If you are working out for less than 450 minutes TOTAL per week consider adding a Sculptor workout AFTER your current workout.

Note: Effective exercise commitment is between 150 and 450 minutes per week.

Weight change D) with measurement outcome 5 – 6

Nutrition and exercise action plans

Your calorie levels, exercise quantity and macronutrient balance are ideal for personal fat loss. Great job. Carry on as you are.

Your calorie levels, exercise quantity and macronutrient balance are ideal for personal fat loss. Great job. Carry on as you are.*

* If you have less than 10 lbs of weight to lose, you should not aim to lose more than 1 lb of weight in any given week. If you have lost more than 1 lb refer to coaching table E) 5-6
If you have less than 5 lbs of weight to lose, you should not aim to lose more than 1/2 lbs of weight in any given week. If you have lost more than 1/2 lb adjust weight accordingly to E) 5-6

The overall focus for group **D)** results is considering your macronutrient balance and some consideration of exercise type. Because you've lost an ideal amount of weight, leave your calories unchanged unless you are having a flux week.

If your weight change was in group **E)** use the following tables to help you make changes for the next week.

Weight change E) with measurement outcome 1- 2

Nutrition action plan

Tracking: Your calorie levels may be too low for long-term fat loss and there is a danger of losing muscle alongside fat. You're doing a great job, but consider increasing your calorie levels by up to 250 kcal per day. Based on your increase in measurements it may also be worth reducing carbohydrates and increasing protein/fat levels.**

Portion control: Your calorie levels are too low for long-term fat loss and there is a danger of losing muscle alongside fat. You're doing a great job, but consider increasing your calorie levels. Based on your increase in measurements it may also be worth reducing carbohydrates and increasing protein/fat levels.**

Intuitive eating: Your calorie levels are too low for long-term fat loss and there is a danger of losing muscle alongside fat. You're doing a great job, but consider increasing your calorie levels. Perhaps it is worth eating a little more than your hunger is telling you that you need.

**Do not reduce carbs lower than 25% of total. Do not increase protein levels to higher than 50% of total.

Exercise action plan

If you are working out for more than 400 minutes TOTAL per week consider removing a resistance or cardio workout from your schedule.

Note: *Effective exercise commitment is between 150 and 450 minutes per week.*

Weight change E) with measurement outcome 3 – 4

Nutrition action plan

Tracking: Your calorie levels are too low for long-term fat loss. You're doing a great job, but consider increasing your calorie levels by up to 250 kcal per day. Based on your measurements it may be worth reducing carbohydrates and increasing protein/fat levels.**

Portion control: Your calorie levels are too low for long-term fat loss and there is a danger of losing muscle alongside fat. You're doing a great job, but consider increasing your portion sizes. Based on your measurements it may also be worth reducing carbohydrates and increasing protein/fat levels. **

Intuitive eating: Your calorie levels are too low for long-term fat loss and there is a danger of losing muscle alongside fat. Perhaps it is worth eating a little more than your hunger is telling you that you need. Based on your measurements it may also be worth reducing carbohydrates and increasing protein/fat levels. **

**Do not reduce carbs lower than 25% of total. Do not increase protein levels to higher than 50% of total.

Exercise action plan

If you are working out for more than 400 minutes TOTAL per week consider removing a resistance or cardio workout from your schedule.

Note: *Effective exercise range is between 150 and 450 minutes per week.*

Weight change E) with measurement outcome 5 – 6

Nutrition action plan

Tracking: Your calorie levels are too low for long-term fat loss. You're doing a great job, but consider increasing your calorie levels by up to 250 kcal per day to ensure you are not losing any muscle further down the line.

Portion control: Your calorie levels are too low for long-term fat loss and there is a danger of losing muscle alongside fat. You're doing a great job, but consider increasing your portion sizes.

Intuitive eating: Your calorie levels are too low for long-term fat loss and there is a danger of losing muscle alongside fat. Perhaps it is worth eating a little more than your hunger is telling you that you need.

Exercise action plan

If you are working out for more than 400 minutes TOTAL per week consider removing a resistance or cardio workout from your schedule.

Note: *Effective exercise range is between 150 and 450 minutes per week.*

The overall focus of change for **E)** is considering increasing your calories to prevent muscle loss alongside potentially looking at your macronutrient balance and some consideration of exercise.

Rationale

Increase carbs: Your calories are too low and your body is possibly using protein for energy via a process called gluconeogenesis. By adding carbs you free up your protein intake to be used for repair.

Decrease carbs: Usually the best macronutrient to recommend dropping for weight loss provided levels are not already low. Nearly always the best macronutrient to drop when weight has been lost but measurements are not dropping. This would normally happen alongside an increase in protein.

Add resistance: When weight has stayed the same or correct weight has been lost, no loss in measurements would indicate muscle could be getting lost. Would nearly always be recommended with an accompanying increase in protein ratios.

Add cardio: Added when calories are not in a deficit. Often a better option than dropping calories if exercise levels are not yet too high and calories are getting too low.

Increase protein: Usually recommended when additional resistance is added and/or when muscle is possibly being lost.

Increase NEAT: Recommended when calories balance is not in a deficit and weight loss is the goal. Increased NEAT can have a significant difference on your metabolism.

Using the analysis charts on a bi-weekly basis

Every two weeks you should refer back to the analysis charts and make changes based on the average outcome of the previous two weeks.

Example 1:

- You lose 2 kg (4.4 lb) on week 1 and 0 kg on week 2
- This is an average of 1 kg (2.2 lb) weight loss (D)

Example 2:

- You lose 1 kg (2.2 lb) on week 1 and gain 1 kg (2.2 lb) on week 2
- This is a balance (C)

Since you only take measurements every two weeks you use the bi-weekly measurement compared with the measurement from two weeks earlier. The analysis charts will enable you to make a decision every two weeks based on the results you have achieved.

General 'self-coaching' principles

The hard part of coaching is tracking data.

Provided you accurately track and measure, the coaching part is remarkably simple. The coaching tables opposite provide *The Blueprint* changes based on the changes to your measurements:

- Calories up and down
- Quantity of exercise
- Protein levels up and down
- Carbohydrate levels up and down

The coaching method has many more variables that you can manipulate, and subtle changes that you can activate to make significant changes.

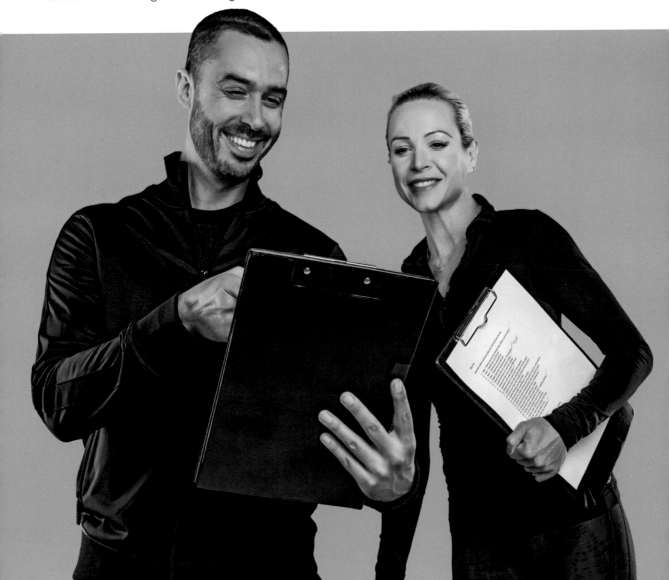

The table below provides a simple idea of changes you can make to your variables based on your goals, compliance and outcomes:

	Healthy eating food ratio	Compliance ratio	Fats	Carbohydrates	Protein	Resistance training	Cardio training	Total exercise	Daily flux ratio	Weekly flux ratio	Calories	NEAT
Gained weight	↓	↓	↑	↑	↑	↓	↑	↓	↑	↑	↑	↓
Lost too much weight			↓	↓	↓	↑	↑	↓	↓	↓	↓	↑
Lost muscle In a deficit	↓	↓			↓	↓			↓	↓	↓	
Lost muscle In a surplus	↓	↓			↓	↓	↓					
Struggling with compliance	↑	↑						↓	↓	↓	↓	
Struggling with energy				↓		↑	↑	↓	↓	↓	↓	
Struggling with cravings	↑	↑		↓	↓				↓	↓	↓	
Performance suffering				↓			↑	↓			↓	
Not enjoying diet	↑	↑							↓	↓		
No weight loss	↓	↓		↑	↓	↓	↓	↓	↑	↑	↑	↓

Further coaching guidelines

Gained weight

If you have gained weight:

- Increase your compliance ratio
- Increase your healthy eating ratio
- Decrease total macronutrients and calories
- Increase your training
- Increase your NEAT

Lost too much weight

If you have lost more than 2 lb (0.9 kg) (consistently – a one-off is not relevant):

- Increase your macronutrients and calories
- Decrease your training/NEAT
- Increase your flux

Lost muscle while in a calorie deficit

If you have lost muscle in an overall deficit there are a number of factors you can consider:

- Increasing your ratio of healthy foods
- Increasing your overall compliance
- Increasing protein
- Increasing resistance training
- Increasing calories
- Increasing the amount of flux days

Lost muscle while in a calorie surplus

If you have lost muscle in an overall surplus there are a number of factors you can consider:

- Increasing your ratio of healthy foods
- Increasing your overall compliance
- Increasing protein (if not already above 40%)
- Increasing resistance training

Struggling with compliance

If you are struggling to stick with your plan you can:

- Decrease your healthy foods ratio
- Decrease your compliance ratio
- Reduce your total exercise
- Introduce more flux

If you are struggling with energy in your plan

Low energy is not a good thing and could be an indication that the training is too high or the calories are too low:

- Increase carbohydrates
- Increase your total calories slightly
- Introduce more frequent flux days to replenish the stocks
- Reduce overall exercise

If your performance is suffering

When performance is suffering it is usually either overtraining, low calories or low carbohydrates:

- Increase carbohydrate ratios
- Reduce total exercise
- Increase flux ratios
- Increase total carbohydrates

If you are not enjoying your diet

Changing the types of foods you eat would be a good start, but in terms of changes you can:

- Decrease healthy ratios
- Decrease overall compliance
- Introduce more flux

If you are not losing any weight

Weight loss is always down to calorie balance, but poor compliance or healthy food ratios can impact the choices you make:

- Increase exercise
- Decrease calories
- Increase compliance
- Increase healthy food ratios
- Increase NEAT

Guidelines on general self coaching principles

1. Don't change too many things at once

Change one, or at most two things at once. If you increase protein, cut carbohydrates, reduce calories, increase exercise and change exercise ratios you won't know which factor made the difference.

2. Make small but significant changes

The bigger the change you make, the less space you have to break plateaus in the future. If your carbohydrates are 40%, don't drop them to 25%, go for 30-35%. If your calories are 1,800, don't go for 1,200, go to 1,600. If you increase your resistance training add ten-minute plug-on workouts or replace one cardio workout. Don't remove all cardio and use only resistance.

3. Be patient and don't panic

Whenever you make a change it may take more than two weeks to see a difference, don't jump to conclusions if things don't improve immediately.

4. Creating your *Blueprint* is central

More important than weight and fat loss is developing an understanding around:

- How many calories your body needs to survive and lose weight
- Which macronutrients your body responds best to
- Which types of exercise make the most difference
- Which exercise and foods you enjoy the most
- Which system is the easiest for you to comply with
- Cravings, emotional eating and hunger control

This is not a super quick-fix process. It takes time and tracking.

Coaching is 95% keeping a track of what you are doing and 5% making the changes.

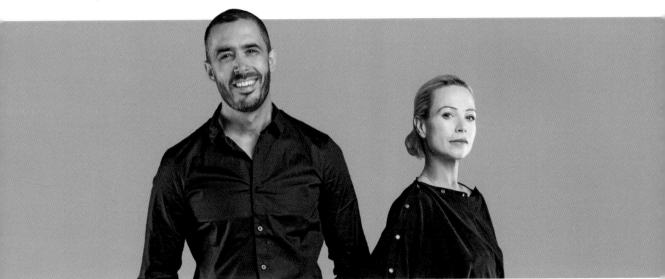

MANAGING EXPECTATION

The basic process of coaching change has just been covered in *The Plan: Analysis of Outcomes*. This framework is the one I have used to help people get in shape for life, for sporting events and everything in between. This process will help you 95% of the time.

Sometimes the results you achieve may not be in line with your expectations or the plan you set yourself is unrealistic. In this instance it is important to reset your expectations or your plan to avoid giving up altogether – the worst case scenario.

Expectation and compliance

It is not uncommon to see the majority of people choose 95% healthy ratios for faster results at the beginning of a health journey before realizing one of two things:

1. The results aren't as fast as they had hoped for.

There is nothing in our advice that will ever move you to faster results than an average of 2 lb (0.9 kg) a week. That is over 100 lb (45 kg) weight loss in a year.

Some people become frustrated at the speed we recommend but this is the best way to retain muscle, lose fat and sustain results.

Provided you are moving forwards you are winning.

2. The expectations you placed on yourself were unrealistic.

'All or nothing' is the fearsome opponent on your journey.

You may find the levels of compliance, exercise and healthy eating are proving unrealistic a while into your health journey. This is both normal and representative of a fork in the road.

You can either:

    A.   Give up and wait until you become frustrated enough to start again.
    B.   Reassess your balance of healthy eating and exercise and create a more realistic plan.

Reassessing your health plan is a very easy thing to do:

- Update your exercise quantity
- Update your healthy/unhealthy eating ratios
- Update your calories
- Update your macronutrients

Provided you choose **b** you will still achieve your desired results. It is important to adapt your plan based on your compliance capability every now and then.

Shifting focus

What do you do at Christmas or during feasts?
What do you do when you go on holiday?
What do you do when you have a particularly busy period of work?
What do you do on a birthday or special occasion?

The answer: Shift focus.

Not meeting personal expectations is why these periods turn into unnecessary failures when our training and nutrition suffers. It is expected and even normal to stop making progress and even lose a little ground at certain times of the year.

Rather than placing unrealistic expectations on yourself, adjust your focus:

- Decide how much exercise you will do in busy periods.
- Decide how much you will relax your nutrition. It is never a good idea to eat unhealthy 100% of the time, but down to 50% over a week is not a problem as a one off.
- Align your behaviours with your expectations. Gaining a couple of pounds is not a problem if it means you can enjoy yourself or get through a busy period.
- Have an inflexible return date. When the fun/busy time is done. Stop.
  Bring your focus back to your long-term goals. It will be hard and it will need discipline but it is crucial for the lifetime of health you want.

The mistake people make is not having a realistic plan for both enjoying holiday times and managing busy times. Be realistic but firm on your return times. If you are realistic with the expectations you place on yourself and the results you achieve, you can continue making progress in perpetuity.

Vicky, 32, England

In the past, every time I have been 'good' and then a special occasion has come along, it's sent me into a tail spin. The last time was my birthday in July, which turned into about 2 weeks of eating rubbish everyday! I fell off the wagon. But 'Transform for Life' has taught me there is no wagon!

So the upcoming celebration of my husband's birthday is being faced differently. Daniel said "Decide if you want to carry on losing weight this week and if you do, make sure you enjoy the celebration, eat and drink as you like, just make up for it elsewhere; cut out snacks, have a fasting period or up the exercise".

I decided to lose the snacks. Ben and I booked my mum to babysit on Friday lunch time.

We went to a beautiful restaurant, it was a lovely occasion. We got dressed up, we had a starter, main and dessert. I had a glass of wine. Ok, two! And a milky latte. I didn't consider the calorie content of anything. It was lovely and memorable. I was so full I didn't even eat any dinner, I just wasn't hungry. I enjoyed every mouthful. Awesome trade for a week of snacks!

And, most importantly, I got straight back onto my plan the following day.

This has been the biggest victory of mindset for me in the process so far. The celebration was lovely. And then I went back to normal. It didn't descend into madness! And if I didn't lose weight this week, that's fine because special occasions are just that, special! They don't happen every week. I'm trusting myself a little more.

IMPORTANT UNDERREPORTING

The reason we recommend calorie flux is less to do with weight loss and more to do with fat loss and muscle retention.

Weight loss and fat loss must be separated in the overall context of calorie flux. If weight loss were the only goal, calorie flux, while still important, would not be as crucial to results.

For the vast majority of people, the reason they aren't losing weight has nothing to do with downregulated metabolisms, carb adaptation, insulin or type of exercise – all of these impact **body composition** more than weight.

Weight loss will always be driven by calorie balance.

A damaged and chronically abused metabolism may show signs of poor insulin response, poor energy distribution, poor glucagon release and any number of issues that are bad for body composition and overall health. None of these are positive for fat loss and health, but none will have a considerable impact on weight loss either.

At its lowest point, a slower metabolism will be anywhere from 100 to 300* kcal lower than its strongest point (based on stable muscle quantity). When we *Reverse diet* (a process of increasing calories without gaining weight, covered later in this section) we are trying to build the metabolism back up by up to 300 kcal, or to its strongest point based on current muscle mass and total body weight.

*NEAT has much higher impact on metabolism.

While a downregulated metabolism would explain slow weight loss with minimal ratio of fat loss, it would not explain why no weight loss occurred at all.

In this instance we can often assume **underreporting** of caloric intake.

Underreporting was the bane of my life as a coach. It made it impossibly hard to provide the correct guidance and we could waste weeks of hard work on both sides alongside potentially detrimental and unnecessary decisions. Before you leap into thinking you have a downregulated metabolism or need to *Reverse diet*, take a while to consider the accuracy of your reporting.

Whether you are estimating intake, writing it down or tracking it through *MyFitnessPal*, take extra care to consider whether you are accurately reporting your total calorie intake.

The biggest areas people don't report or underreport are:

- Oils added to food
- Butter added to food
- Picking food off other people's plates
- Eating while cooking
- Milk, cream and sugar in teas and coffees
- Dressings
- Sauces

Studies have found people to be underreporting by 1,000 kcal per day or more based on the above factors!

The more accurate you are with your reporting, the easier you will find managing your overall results and outcomes.

To weigh or not to weigh

When it come to tracking food, the question of whether to weigh food often comes up, and this is a relevant discussion in the context of this chapter.

Weighing Calories

I was working with a client who felt it important to reduce calories further as she had stopped losing weight at 1400 kcal.

Looking at her food data, I noticed she was eating around 100g of carbohydrates every evening (rice, pasta or potato).

As she was already eating just 1400 kcal daily, I was reluctant to drop calories further, feeling it was unlikely she wasn't losing weight with such low calories and high quantities of exercise.

So rather than reduce calories further, I asked her to start weighing calories in her evening meals - a relatively extreme measure for some, but not nearly as extreme as asking her to reduce calories to a level I felt uncomfortable with.

After just one night she came back to me.

"I really thought I was eating around 100g of rice, it turns out I was eating 200g."
This was a difference of 400 calories.

She started weighing her food and we INCREASED her calories to 1600 kcal, a level at which she started losing weight.

I experienced many scenarios similar to this one over the years.

Does this mean you should weigh food?

I don't think weighing everything is always important (although some coaches will disagree) but I do think spending time weighing when you **start tracking** is a good idea to ensure you are able to correctly gauge quantities.

Estimating quantity in foods when you first start tracking is nigh on impossible without experience - with experience you can be accurate with your estimates without the need for weighing.

Like everything with *Transform for Life*, the hard work is put in upfront when learning - the process becomes gradually easier the longer you go.

Dry weight or cooked weight?

Do you calculate your foods based on the cooked weight or the raw weight?

Overall I would opt for the raw, uncooked weight if possible.

General rule:

- Carbohydrates normally become heavier during cooking through soaking up water up
- Proteins will normally become lighter during cooker through releasing water

Example: Chicken Breast

100 gram serving of chicken breast can shrink to 80 grams or less!

Example: Rice

If you cook rice in 2 cup of water vs 4 cups of water, absorption of water creates a higher weight in the rice cooked in 4 cups.

This is why uncooked is usually better.

There is never a perfect solution. When tracking food, it is important to take as many factors as you can into account and then provide your best estimate.

Eating out, eating at friends and other factors will make it impossible to ever be 100% accurate, but the more you track, the better you will become at accurately estimating how much food you are eating.

After several weeks your intuition will point you in the right direction 99% of the time.

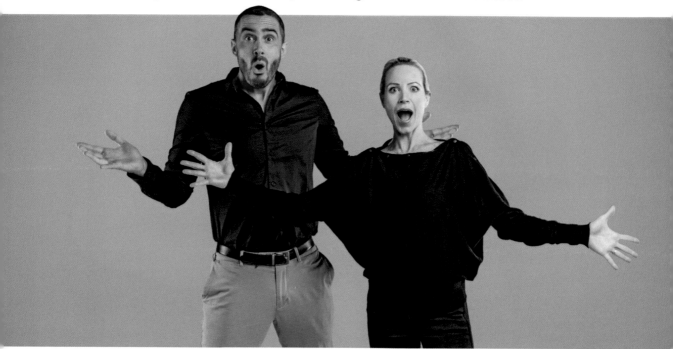

EXERCISE ACCELERATORS

If you have met with a plateau and your exercise is not in excess of 450 minutes per week you could introduce accelerators to push results on.

Whenever you increase exercise levels beyond your sustainable long-term habits, it is important you identify for how long and for what purpose you are doing it.

An exercise accelerator is placed in category E below and should not be confused with your baseline habit of A.

Habit types

A. Sustainable healthy habit – a daily occurrence that becomes part of life. This should be the main focus of any health plan (daily workout, eating vegetables, drinking water, portion management, walking).

B. Consistent unhealthy habit – a daily occurrence that damages long-term results. Removing these should be the main focus of any health plan (daily junk food, sedentary behaviour, emotional eating).

C. Planned unhealthy habit – a regular habit that is part of your plan. Yes PART OF YOUR PLAN. YOU decide when and how often you eat 'unhealthy' foods, kick back on the couch, have a glass of wine, etc. This is an important part of any long-term health plan.

D. Decelerator – a one off, undesirable behaviour where impact is overestimated. It will actually have little impact if a one off. Stopping it becoming a consistent unhealthy habit is the key (missing a workout, giving in to a craving and eating a cake, etc).

E. Conscious accelerator – a planned, healthy behaviour that is understood to not be sustainable, but is implemented in the short-term to accelerate results (double workout, lowering carb intake, removing planned unhealthy habit).

F. Unconscious accelerator – a behaviour that is seen to be positive but is entirely unsustainable (super low-carb diet, unsustainable total abstinence, overtraining). These are dangerous behaviours that often result in rebound behaviours.

Sculptors

Sculptors are 10-15 minute plug-ons that are designed to add to your workout plan. This additional work will result in a small calorie burn increase, but greater protein synthesis and superior muscle adaptation.

The increased demand for protein as a 'repair' substrate will place additional pressure on the body to 'free' stored fat for energy alongside positively rebuilding the muscles worked.

The complete Sculptors guide is available for all members at:

www.teambodyproject.com/additional-resources

Turbos

Turbos have a variety of guises with benefits dependent on the type of *Turbo* workout you do. You can learn more about *Turbos* in the *The Exercise Handbook* in *Additional Resources*. The additional calories burned with a *Turbo* mean you can retain calorie levels and create a further deficit.

Note: *Both Sculptors and Turbos are focused exercise that breaks down muscle tissue. For this reason we do not recommend more than 450 minutes a week.*

NEAT

The wonderful thing about NEAT (Non-exercise activity thermogenesis) or how many steps we walk and how much we move in general, is that it is not catabolic (breaking down tissue) in the same way focused exercise is. Therefore a reasonable increase in our activity offers benefits to our calorie balance without risk of overtraining.

Buying a pedometer or tracking steps using your phone (there are many free apps) would be an excellent addition. You can set yourself a short-term target of steps and focus on walking that far every day.

Note: *We should always focus on an absolute minimum of 5,000 steps. You can gauge your current movement levels by tracking your steps before you introduce an accelerator.*

Accelerators would start at an additional 2,500 steps and upwards.

Steps as 'accelerators'

Example 1:
5,000 steps = current baseline steps being taken
5,000 steps = additional accelerator steps
10,000 steps = short-term steps target

Example 2:
7,500 steps = current baseline steps being taken
2,500 steps = additional accelerator steps
10,000 steps = short-term steps target

Example 3:
10,000 steps = current baseline steps being taken
7,500 steps = additional accelerator steps
17,500 steps = short-term steps target

THE PERSONAL COMPLIANCE CHART

Type	What it is	How often?
Obsession	Every action you take, every food you eat and every moment of your day revolves around what you eat, when you train and what you look like. This is NOT good.	0%
Dedication	You have a very clear goal and you intend to hit it. You are willing to make sacrifices and serious short-term changes to your diet and exercise in order to make it happen. (Never confuse dedication with obsession. Dedication is an admirable application to a goal.)	5-20%
Consistency	You have a balanced goal to make progress in the context of everything else in your life. You let little things go and think about the long-term. You are consistent with your training and nutrition as part of your life and understand that you can't just 'do what you want' if you want a desirable outcome. **Note:** *This is where 90% of progress is made and where we want most of you!*	60-90%
Loose compliance	You are not showing any strong consistency or direction with your plan. You are eating mostly what you feel like while keeping an eye on not letting it get out of control. You tend to train when you feel like it. This is 100% better than non-compliance but can't be expected to generate any visible results (although 'unseen' results are plenty). It will hold you together during difficult times.	10-40%
Non-compliance	It is what it is. You eat what you like and stop training. We don't want to go here!	0%

Your goal should be to stay between 'dedication' and 'consistency', stay out of 'obsession' and 'non-compliance' and entering loose compliance in challenging periods and times of maintenance.

'Non-compliance' and 'obsession' are the Richard Burton and Elizabeth Taylor or Bonnie and Clyde of the workout world...

... Dangerously drawn to one another!

Exercise compliance versus nutrition compliance

Having exercise in 'dedication' and nutrition in 'loose compliance' does not equal consistency. Overall results will be led by the nutrition factor. So if you have training in 'dedication' but nutrition in 'loose compliance' total results will more likely be led by 'loose compliance'.

Quality of results will be driven by the exercise factor. If you have nutrition in 'dedication' but exercise in 'non-compliance', you can't expect fat loss and muscle retention, just weight loss. Your quality of body composition will be driven by the exercise factor!

Compliance questions and answers

If you are feeling miserable or tired while trying to lose fat, you need to consider if you are following a sustainable long-term solution for you. Whenever you are feeling this way, you need to ask yourself a few questions.

1. Is my current nutrition and exercise plan in line with my long-term sustainability plan?

Yes. We all have different levels of personal compliance capability. Consider whether your calorie balance, your macronutrient intake, your flux and your healthy/unhealthy balance is sustainable and make changes.

No. How long are you intending to accelerate your results with short-term habits? There is never any harm in dropping off to a more sustainable pace if you are finding your current levels too much.

2. I am missing 'naughty' treats and snacks. What can I do?

Provided you eat a predominantly healthy diet, there is no issue with having a treat for a snack. In the context of an overall healthy diet, a small 100 kcal chocolate bar is going to make no greater difference to your body composition than 100 kcal worth of nuts. The question is, are you ready to introduce 'naughty' snacks?

Yes you are. The 'naughty' snack itches the scratch and helps you adhere to your diet.

No you are not. The 'naughty' snack fires off a chain reaction of cravings and an insatiable desire for more of the same.

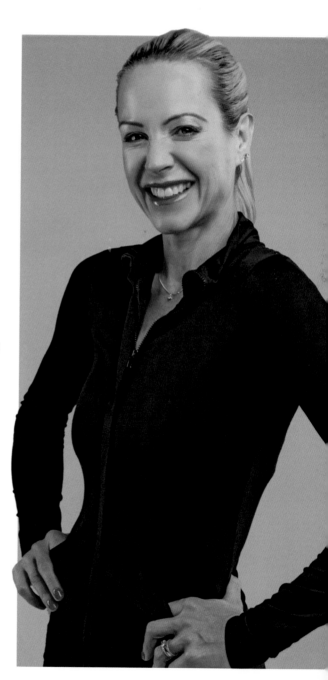

3. I am feeling miserable, tired and hungry and yet I am barely losing any weight. I cannot face dropping my calories any further. What can I do?

It may be time to rebuild your metabolism and change your focus. If you're feeling this way now, there is no way you can sustain this for the long-term.

Note: *Read our upcoming chapter on Reverse Dieting (pages 240-242).*

FURTHER INDIVIDUALIZATION

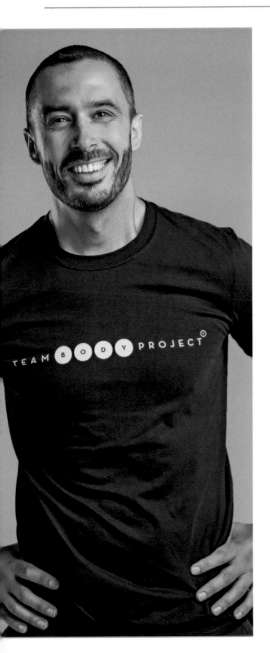

If you have been following the coaching guidelines, making adaptations to your program and being compliant but have still stopped making the progress you want, it is worth considering further individualization.

It is very unlikely you will need to introduce any of the methods in this chapter if:

- You have been training for less than six months
- You have more than 10 lb (4.5 kg) in total body weight to lose

Before you try any further individualization methods you should read and follow these chapters:

- *Underreporting (discussed earlier in The Bluprint)*
- *Ten Basic Compliance Principles (Additional Resources)*

If you have exhausted other paths and still need a fresh approach, the following methods are useful for making further progress or repairing poor metabolic processes:

- Fasting
- Carb cycling
- Nutrient timing
- Reverse dieting

FASTING

If you want to lose weight while maximizing fat loss and retaining muscle, the headline acts will always be calorie balance, exercise, macronutrient balance, quality of food and avoiding chronic exposure to extreme measures. Fasting, or any other method beyond this, is only as effective as your capacity to adhere to these basic rules.

If you fast for 16 hours a day, but don't exercise, eat a caloric surplus and eat processed foods composed of 90% carbohydrates, the fasting itself won't do much good for you. That being said, I have found fasting to be specifically useful in two ways:

1. To give people a simple, short-term way of breaking a plateau without causing metabolic damage.

2. To help people that are too busy to prepare three plus meals or more a day, or struggle with counting calories and other tracking methods, to reduce calories.

Fasting is not our standard approach. There will be far more detailed resources available to you if you wish to pursue it as a long-term strategy, however, this guide should help you decide whether fasting is a possible protocol to achieve your own goals.

Note: *I will not be approaching the research on whether intermittent fasting has 'longevity' benefits, but rather considering it alongside our goal of long-term, sustainable health behaviours and healthy weight results.*

What is intermittent fasting?

Intermittent fasting is fasting applied intermittently. It is the opposite of the 'little and often' approach since it is more focused on longer periods without food alongside larger portions.

We could call fasting 'more food, less often'.

This 'more food, less often' approach could be skipping one meal a day, having whole days with no meals or any number of varying durations of 'fast' and 'feast' in between.

There are three main ways people approach fasting:

1. **Meal skipping**
   Skip a predetermined number of meals in a week with the ultimate goal of eating fewer calories. Example: Skip breakfast every day.

2. **Total day fasting**
   Limit your calories to approximately 500 kcal on fasting days and avoid exercise on these days.

3. **Shrink the eating window**
   Reverse the amount of time in your day to include eight hours of eating time and 16 hours of fasting time (usually paired with specific exercise-led nutrient timing and fasted cardio). We find this method the most complicated and hardest to comply with and therefore are not covering it in further detail in this book.

Fasting as a long-term strategy

Net calorie deficit, macronutrient balance, regular exercise and a predominance of high quality food will always remain the priority for health and long-term weight management.

Despite what some may say, intermittent fasting does not allow you to escape the fundamental rules of health and weight management. There are some who would suggest that, provided you have 'fasting' days, you can eat whatever what you want the rest of the time; but this is not accurate.

Once the baseline of fundamentals is established there is no considerable difference between 'little and often' and intermittent fasting in achieving your goals. (Intermittent fasting-specific factors beyond healthy weight management are not considered here.)

Note: *Different people respond to different methods in different ways. Any physical differences would be seen at an individual level, i.e. some people may respond to one better than another. The only way you will learn how well **you** respond compared to other methods, is by doing it.*

The initial choice as to whether intermittent fasting is right for you is best based on the following factors:

- Whether it is easier for you to implement within your lifestyle and circumstances
- Whether you find it easier to miss meals than count calories or track portions (long-term)
- Whether you find fasting easier to comply with long-term than other methods of weight management

Before you jump on the fasting train I do want you to consider the following...

In a long career of coaching people to lose weight, a large majority of people I worked with were skipping breakfast. In other words, they were already applying an intermittent fasting strategy. In most of these cases they weren't losing weight and in many cases they were gaining weight, which is usually why they came to see me.

Fasting was causing them to make poor food choices later in the day and overeat. There is no benefit to skipping a meal, if skipping a meal causes you to make progressively worse choices throughout the day. Therefore, effective fasting can only be implemented from a known point of balance; for example, once you understand the size and frequency of meals and snacks your body needs daily to maintain calorie balance.

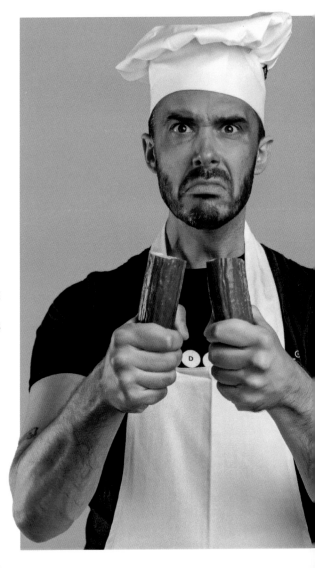

- Intermittent fasting can be utilized by removing meals or snacks to create caloric deficits
- Intermittent fasting can be utilized by implementing total fasting days to create caloric deficits

If you are fasting to lose weight, having a fasting day does not allow for overeating on days when you are not fasting. This would create a balance or an imbalance, rather than a deficit.

Fasting does not allow us to circumvent the laws of thermodynamics, it simply provides us with a different method of creating calorie balances and imbalances.

I see the specific benefits of fasting to be more closely aligned with improved hunger reading, craving control and discipline development. Overall, whether fasting works for you is a combination of psychological and physiological factors laid against the overall desire of optimal body composition.

Try it alongside the key principles to find out if it works for you.

Fasting for busting a plateau

Fasting is a positive thing for most people to try every once in awhile. Everybody should consider attempting it at least once if there are no medical contraindications.

There are a few unique benefits to fasting beyond caloric reduction:

- It teaches discipline
- You learn hunger management
- It develops craving control
- It helps us understand the difference between physical hunger (body hunger) and psychological hunger (appetite)

A fasting day once or twice a week when you are experiencing a plateau can provide the additional reduction to your caloric deficit to kickstart your weight loss without damage to your metabolism.

When trying to lose weight, chronic exposure to any extreme measure is the most important thing to avoid. Chronic exposure to daily deficits – low carbs, high protein diets and any other chronic exposures – creates an environment for reduced metabolic function and flexibility.

A fasting day introduced occasionally as a one-off or even a series of one-offs will have positive impacts on your body composition without negative impacts on your metabolism.

Conclusions

Overall, I do not see strong research that suggests fasting is a better dietary strategy than frequent eating, or visa versa. The majority of benefits you take from both fasting and smaller frequent meals are due to a lower calorie diet and (hopefully) a reduction in processed foods.

While the specific outcomes may come via different physiological pathways, the outcomes are similar enough to warrant both as a potential approach. For this reason, the choice as to whether fasting is right for you should be more compliance-led than anything else.

1. Trying fasting is a great way to practise 'hunger management' and this is a very important tool for everybody looking to manage weight.

2. Fasting is not any better (or worse) for losing body fat. It could be a more practical or easier method for you to implement, but it will not produce objectively better or worse fat-loss results than similar caloric deficits created with frequent meals.

3. It can be a good approach for people who are very busy and people who really don't like counting calories. Once you know your personal 'homeostasis' point you can create deficits with the removal of meals.

This is an easier strategy for some than counting calories, but it shouldn't be approached without some form of *Blueprint* creation.

4. Food quality remains important if you want to implement fasting. Just because you have fasted doesn't mean you can eat whatever you want.

5. Whatever you choose, effective fat-loss with muscle retention will always come back to Lily's Laws.

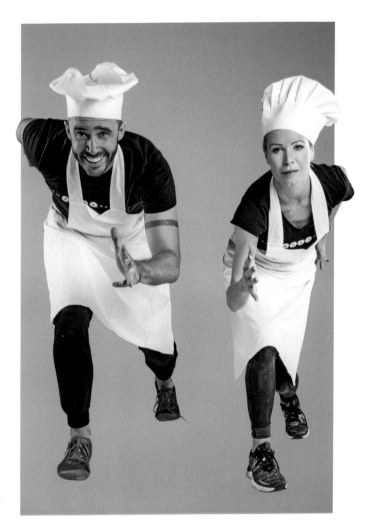

Lily's Laws

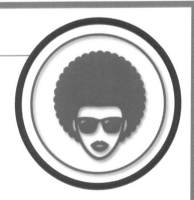

Lily wanted to pop by to remind us that nutrition is a vital component to change.

- Calorie balance
- Anabolic and catabolic flux
- Sufficient carbohydrates
- Sufficient protein
- Sufficient fat
- Drink enough water
- Eat plenty of vegetables
- Limit processed food intake
- Exercise to stimulate muscle growth and fat loss
- NEAT is an important aspect of your metabolic rate

CARB CYCLING

Carb cycling is a very low carbohydrate (and usually calorie) diet, with intermittent 'refeeds' of higher calorie and carbohydrate days.

I do not see any reason why anybody who has reasonable goals, has patience and is persistent will ever have to take on heavy carb cycling. I have included this to ensure that those who use this method do so correctly and safely.

This is not a healthy lifestyle plan, it is an aesthetic plan. There should be a degree of flux in all diets.

Note 1: *I am not a fan of this strategy. I believe in sustainability at the top of any health plan, but unlike many coaches I do not believe my opinion matters. If you want to have visible abs and are willing to pay the price, it is your choice, and this is proven to be an effective strategy.*

Note 2: *This strategy is entirely unnecessary and surplus to requirements if you have more than 10% of body weight to lose.*

Aggressive calorie/carb cycling

I have used very low carb diets that included cycled 'refeeds' with individuals who suit the approach and understand the implications, but it is only an effective strategy when based on the following:

1. It is not a long-term protocol
2. You do not have an 'all or nothing' mindset (it holds a high level of danger for rebound)
3. You have a high tolerance for compliance
4. You can handle very low carb/calorie diets
5. You are not vegetarian or vegan
6. You can tolerate hunger and cravings very well
7. You do not have a history of yo-yo dieting

Guidelines:

1. Drop carbohydrates to around 15% for 7-14 days at a time. This usually means entirely cutting out all starchy carbs and even limiting fruit.
2. Calories should be around 30% lower than current baseline.
3. Increase high protein, high fat based foods (meats, oily fish, eggs).
4. Eat A LOT of leafy green vegetables.
5. Show additional caution to cheese, nuts, milk and oils.
6. Constantly remind yourself that a 'refeed' is coming.
7. Every 7 to 14 days have a 'refeed' day. On this day you will significantly increase your carbohydrate levels. You should aim to eat between 2 and 3 times your lower calories on refeed days, with most of the additional calories coming from carbohydrate sources.
8. You should up your training or have your 'hardest' training day on the refeed day to maximize muscle repair and adaptation.

Example: If you are eating 1,200 kcal on low carb days, you should aim for between 2,400 and 3,600 kcal on refeed days, mostly from carb sources. (x 2 for shorter cycles and x 3 for longer cycles).

Theory:
- This refeed is going to stop your body from downregulating metabolic processes
- This would allow you to eat lower than average calories over a weekly or bi-weekly period
- Because of the refeed we prevent the body from converting stored muscle into energy

Let's imagine your normal baseline calorie level is 1,800 kcal and you eat 1,200 kcal daily during the two weeks of aggressive carb cycling:

Carb cycling

Bi-weekly refeed

Normal: 1,800 kcal per day x 14 = 25,200 kcal.
CC: 1,200 kcal per day x 13 + 3,600 refeed kcal = 19,200 kcal

Result:
2 lb (0.9 kg) of additional fat loss (if all else equal)

Weekly refeed

Normal: 1,800 kcal per day x 7 = 12,600 kcal
CC: 1,200 kcal per day x 6 + 3,600 refeed kcal = 10,800 kcal

Result:
0.5-1lb (0.2-0.45 kg) of additional fat loss (if all else equal)

Further to the calorie benefits we would see from carb cycling illustrated on the previous page, it is considered you will experience improved glucagon production.

This is positive in the context of fat loss as glucagon is the hormone responsible for freeing fat stores for energy use.

Final note on carb cycling

This dietary approach should never be used for more than 8-12 weeks, after which a more sustainable and long-term nutrition plan should be returned to.

NUTRIENT TIMING

Nutrient timing is the fuelling of your body with the correct nutrients at suitable times to maximize the processes of change you want your body to undertake. Essentially this is manipulation of food intake before, during and after a workout.

Does nutrient timing matter?

No	Possibly
You have more than 10 lb (4.5 kg) to lose	You have less than 10 lb (4.5 kg) to lose
You are still making reasonable progress	You have stopped making reasonable progress
You exercise for less than 45 minutes at a time	You exercise for more than 45 minutes at a time
You want moderate fat loss	You want less than 10% fat (male), 18% (female)
You don't use fasting	You use fasting

At the top line, the total amount of calories from carbohydrates, fats and proteins is far more important than the timing of them. We should never assume that a detail like nutrient timing can supercede the importance of total nutrient intake.

Hierarchy of importance

1. Amount of calories (total calorie intake)
2. Quality of calories (whole, healthy foods versus processed foods)
3. Macronutrient ratio of calories (protein, fats and carbs)
4. Timing of calories (when you eat the calories)

Methods of nutrient timing:

- Anabolic window
- Fasted cardio

The anabolic window of opportunity takes advantage of short-term benefits like improved protein synthesis and glycogen replenishment, but research does not actually show a huge impact on the long-term advantages we want, like lower fat and higher muscle.

This does not mean it is not important, just that it's not as important as people may think.

Fasted cardio is taking advantage of a fasted state of unavailable dietary nutrients. The production of glucagon alongside the energy requirements of exercise theoretically creates fat mobilization.

The problem is, research shows that fasted cardio works better for some than others and nutrient timing is effective in the short-term but shows minimal long-term benefits.

When we allow nutrient timing to overtake the importance of total nutrient intake we can make mistakes like eating large amounts of highly processed, refined foods in the window of opportunity because we believe we will get away with it.

This does not mean nutrient timing will not make a difference to your results or enable you to break through a plateau. Just that it is not a magic bullet.

With body composition, if you want your body to utilize the nutrients coming in at the time when they are most effective, it makes sense to consume them around the time they are going to be most needed.

The problem is, this varies from person to person. You can try out various methods of nutrient timing, measure against results and see if they make a difference for you without ever forgetting the hierarchy of importance when it comes to good nutrition.

Hierarchy of importance

1.   Amount of calories (total calorie intake)
2.   Quality of calories (whole, healthy foods versus processed foods)
3.   Macronutrient ratio of calories (protein, fats and carbs)
4.   Timing of calories (when you eat the calories)

How to change your nutrient timing

When it comes to nutrient timing, all the research points towards one thing: when you're stuck, a change makes a difference. What that means, in its simplest terms, is to change what you're doing.

- If you're currently eating breakfast before cardio but results have slowed, try doing cardio without eating breakfast first
- If you're currently eating six meals a day, try eating four meals a day
- If you're currently spreading macronutrients evenly across all meals, try loading your carbs after a workout

1. Meal frequency

Six small meals means:

- Constant availability of protein for repair
- Reduced hunger and cravings
- Insulin-dominant environment
- More even energy distribution

Three larger meals means:

- Glucagon-dominant environment
- More cravings and hunger
- Less frequent availability of protein for repair

With other factors being equal, studies show no significant difference, but:

1. People looking to build more muscle may do better with more meals
2. People looking to lose fat may do better with fewer meals

I would recommend changing your meal frequency if:

- You are stuck in a plateau
- It fits your lifestyle
- You have good compliance
- Minimal body fat is important to you

2. Pre- and post-workout carb timing

Carb timing is used to provide carbs for energy and protein synthesis at times when they are specifically needed; for energy during workouts and for anabolic repair.

Proposed benefits of loading carbs before and after a workout:

- Improved protein synthesis
- Better glycogen replenishment
- Improved performance
- Carb quota used on performance

This method is built around the idea of an 'anabolic window of opportunity'.

On the other hand, carb distribution would focus on spreading them through the day.

Proposed benefits of balanced carb distribution:

- Even blood sugar
- Reduced hunger and cravings
- Less potential for muscle breakdown due to gluconeogenesis
- More sustainable

This method is built around the idea of sustainable hunger and craving control and balanced energy throughout the day.

If I were working with an elite athlete, where 2 lb (0.9 kg) of muscle could make the difference between winning and losing, there is no doubt I would choose carb timing. By far the most important factor for an elite-level athlete is performance.

On the other hand, if I were working with a non-professional athlete who wanted to lose fat but also needed carbs to function for other purposes, I would choose carb distribution throughout the day.

I would recommend carb timing for breaking a plateau:

- If you have excellent compliance
- If you can handle cravings
- If you can handle hunger
- If minimal body fat is important to you

REVERSE DIETING

If you have been following our guidelines on sustainable weight loss, hitting points in your health journey where you need to rebuild your metabolism should be avoidable.

However, if you have a history of crash dieting and/or prolonged and extreme carbohydrate reduction it is very possible you will struggle to lose weight with normal calorie reductions and activity level, even when following our guidelines.

If this is the case, you may want to rebuild your metabolism, through a 'reverse dieting' process.

Should I reverse diet?

Whether reverse dieting is right for you should be based on a combination of the following:

1. If you are exercising more than 400 minutes per week.

    AND

2. You have a diet that is:
A. Lower than 1,200 kcal per day as a female
B. Lower than 1,500 kcal per day as a male

These are rough guidelines. I would start showing caution to weight loss sustainability any time you drop below 1,350 kcal as a female and 1,650 kcal as a male, when exercise is in excess of 350 minutes per week.

On the other hand if your exercise is less than 250 minutes a week, even when calories are low, it is possible increasing exercise may be a far better option than reverse dieting in the first instance.

Note: *Stale weight loss is when you have lost 1 lb (0.45 kg) or less (total) in a four week period. Do not assume you need to reverse diet because your weight loss has stopped for a week or even two. This is perfectly normal and even expected at times.*

Reverse dieting

Reverse dieting is typically used for athletes, such as boxers and bodybuilders, to rebuild metabolic rate after periods of extreme caloric reductions and exercise. For reasons I have never completely understood, this well-known technique in sporting circles has never crossed over into mainstream use.

The theory of reverse dieting is not very different to the reason we flux our calories on a regular basis. We move the body slowly out of a chronic hypocaloric state and into a hypercaloric state while either:

A.   Not gaining weight
B.   Gaining a small amount of weight that would be exclusively muscle

Reverse dieting is more of a psychological battle than a physiological one. Training hard to build small amounts of muscle, rather than lose fat, can be hard mentally after many years of trying to lose fat.

To get reverse dieting right requires paying attention to tracking weight and measurements. Our goal is to place the body into an increasingly anabolic state until we raise our metabolism and metabolic processes back to a healthier state.

Once we have established a stronger metabolism, we can begin the process of healthy fat loss again without danger of losing muscle and without the need for extreme restrictions.

How long will it take to rebuild my metabolism?

It depends on a number of factors, including how long you have been exposed to very low calorie diets. It could take as little as a few weeks and as much as several months. While this may feel frustrating, I always remind people of the reason they are reverse dieting. They have stopped losing weight anyway. Many times, people have been stuck at a weight for many months in a low calorie/high exercise state. They have nowhere left to go and if they wish to make further progress this is the only way forwards.

When reverse dieting, progress simply gets measured in a different way.

How it works

Here is a step by step guide to reverse dieting:

It is important you have been tracking calories if you wish to implement this. It can be very difficult to do using other methods without gaining weight.

A.   **Increase the ratio of resistance training in your routine.** The Personal Training workouts, Danger Zone, Superhero, Pure Resistance and Sculptors are all excellent resistance based workouts. This will mean you should reduce the ratio of cardio in your routine accordingly.

B.   **Increase your kcal by 100 per day.** This would normally start with carbohydrates, (usually lowest in chronic dieters). Over time, you should increase across all macronutrients.

Example:
Current diet: Consume 1,000 kcal per day.
New diet: Consume 1,100 kcal per day.

Note: *It really is that simple. Somehow, there are entire books on this subject and yet the process is no more complicated than this.*

C. **Follow the new routine.** For the next seven days, follow your new training routine and diet with higher calories, tracking your consumption.

D. **Remeasure.** At the end of the seven days, weigh and measure yourself.

- **If you weigh the same.** Increase your kcal by 100 again. Repeat.
- **If you have gained weight.** You should stick with your calorie consumption until your weight stabilizes. You can also change your macronutrient ratios*.
- **If you have lost weight.** Increase your kcal by up to 200. You can also change your macronutrient ratios*.

E. Repeat the process every week until you have raised your calorie consumption to a more sustainable long-term quantity. Your goal is to strengthen your metabolism and resume balanced metabolic processes while building muscle.

* I always get asked what the best macronutrient ratio is. Over time you will learn which macronutrient ratios you will respond best to. The only way to know what is best for you is trial and error.

Being in an anabolic state and a caloric surplus is a positive thing for your body.

1. Your body switches on processes it had previously switched off. You will have more energy, better sleep and more positive moods.

2. Your body remembers it can use protein for building muscle, not just for converting into energy for use.

3. Your body may even start to mobilise fat sources it has been holding on to. People find this to be the most surprising benefit.

Patience

Enjoy rebuilding your body and your metabolism, the longer you spend building a healthy body, the faster you will meet your ultimate health goals.

The key word here is building. After a long period of breaking down tissue and fat, you are building health again.

Reverse dieting is over-complicated by many people. It is a simple process of increasing calories, increasing resistance training and tracking changes until you are satisfied with your new point of balance.

Once you are eating a healthy amount of calories, you can start the process of reducing calories and losing fat once again, but this time remembering to introduce regular flux so you don't have to reverse diet again.

CAN A METABOLISM BE 'BROKEN'?

Some people feel that their metabolisms are seriously damaged and that it is impossible to lose weight.

After a lifetime of dieting, it can feel like no matter what you try, you simply can't drop the pounds.

Calorie balance is confusing because it is not always as simple as it seems. As adaptations happen in your body, it can seem like your body is not obeying the laws of physics, but this is a dangerous line of thinking that can lead to extreme or false measures and a mindset that becomes open to seemingly exciting marketing messages that are infused with nonsense.

Regardless of how often you have dieted you will not circumvent thermodynamics and no amount of magic avocados or juice cleanses can change this. Any avoidable adaptations your body has made will be predictable, fixable and not particularly extreme.

Rather than reaching the understandable but false conclusion that your body doesn't work, it is better to understand your body and how it does work, so you can make changes accordingly and in line with your personal goals.

Regardless of how effectively you lose weight there will be:

1. Unavoidable slowing adaptations to your resting metabolic rate (a smaller object requires less energy to survive)

2. A reduction in the amount of calories you burn during exercise (a smaller object requires less energy to be used)

Therefore, if you start losing weight at 1800 kcal and lose 20 lb, you will probably need to reduce your calories to continue losing weight. This is not indicative of a damaged metabolism, this is indicative of success.

A slower metabolism is an inevitable side effect of weighing less, but chronic dieting **can** also cause additional processes to change in your body, making weight loss even harder:

> **1.Thermic effect of eating goes down when you eat less for prolonged periods of time.**
>
> The body will spend less energy on digestion when it doesn't have sufficient calories.
>
> **2. NEAT adapts down when calories are permanently low.**
>
> Your body is a complex machine. With less calories to 'waste' your body will stop wanting to move.
>
> **3. Calories absorbed increases – you absorb more of the calories you eat.**
>
> Calorie absorption will increase when you are in a permanent calorie deficit. This may mean that where you were absorbing 1500 per 2000 kcal consumed before reducing calories, your body may now be absorbing 1800 per 2000 kcal consumed.

What does all this mean?

Your body is certainly not broken.

It uses less energy to digest food because it is reluctant to waste calories. It is hesitant to move more because it doesn't want to burn and waste calories, and it is absorbing a higher percentage of the food you consume because it doesn't want to waste calories.

Some people call this 'starvation mode' when in reality it is just the body being understandably more prudent with calorie expenditure when there are fewer calories available.

Let's compare two people that weigh 200 lb to illustrate what dieting can do:

	Person 1 – always weighed 200 lb	Person 2 – Dieted down from 250 lb
Weight	200 lb	200 lb
Daily calorie intake	2000 kcal	2000 kcal
Actual Calorie absorption	90% (2000 x 0.8) 1800 kcal	95% (2000 x 0.95) 1900 kcal
Resting metabolic rate (RMR)	1200 kcal	1200 kcal
Natural NEAT	450 kcal per day	350 kcal per day
Thermic impact	5% (2000 x 0.05) 200 kcal	2.5% (2000 x 0.025) 100 kcal
Daily workout	250 kcal	250 kcal
Daily calorie balance	300 kcal (weight loss)	0 kcal (weight maintenance)

* Results in this table are demonstrative values only and actual figures could be very different

The RMR and daily workout figures are identical to one another since a lower weight inevitably reduces RMR and calories burned during a workout.

Note: *the RMR could vary by up to 15%, but this is largely genetic and out of our control.*

However, adaptive NEAT, thermogenesis and calorie absorption make the difference in outcomes rather noticeable.

It is **very likely** that somebody who has lost weight will not be able to exist on the same amount of calories as somebody who weighs the same as them, but has retained this weight for a long period of time.

Add to this the 15% difference in RMR that can exist from person to person, and if you're on the lower end of RMR, it really can feel like the world is against you when trying to lose weight.

However, please remember this: Everybody loses weight in a calorie deficit.

What is NOT happening:

1. You are **not** eating less than 1200 kcal per day and still not losing weight (unless you weigh less than 100 lb and even then you would need to be sedentary). Your body will retain a relatively stable RMR regardless of how much you diet. If you think you are eating 1200 kcal, exercising for an hour a day and still not losing weight you are probably **vastly** miscalculating the amount of food you are eating. (See the chapter on *Underreporting*)

2. Your body is **not** seriously damaged by a lifetime of dieting. It has made some inevitable adaptations alongside some fixable adaptations that make losing weight more challenging. Losing weight can be hard, but we are here to support you.

3. You are **not** defying the laws of thermodynamics. You can lose weight if you create an imbalance, everybody can. Calorie balance is not as simple as 'calories in versus calories out' (as illustrated above) but it is never, ever false.

What can be done?

1. **Calorie flux**

Avoid staying in permanent calorie deficits to minimise the impact of adaptive processes when losing weight.

Flux protects our metabolism from adaptive processes and allows us to build muscle, which is more metabolically active than fat.

2. **Accept the facts**

Your metabolic rate is your metabolic rate, it is not your fault and your body is not broken! Your metabolism may not be as you wish it to be, but only a small part of that is within our control. It is possible that another person with most of the same factors as you can lose weight at 2000 kcal and for you to lose weight you must consume 1500 kcal. This may not be fair, but if you want results it must be accepted. If you are not losing weight and you wish to, you are eating too many calories for weight loss. You may not think you are eating too many calories, but you are.

Note: *If you are seriously concerned about your metabolic rate and are eating less than 1200 kcal a day alongside regular exercise and not losing weight, this needs investigation beyond the scope of this book. Contact your doctor or physician to discuss further.*

3. **Consider food quality**

Processed foods have a much higher absorption rate than non processed foods. They also have a lower thermic effect. The increased processes required to digest fibre, nutrient rich foods means we spend more energy digesting them and absorb less of the calories in the process.

4. **Reverse diet**

Increasing calories while sustaining weight will slowly support increased NEAT, decreased absorption and increased thermic effect.

5. **Monitor NEAT**

Your body may not want to move as much when you are in a calorie deficit, but that doesn't mean it can't move as much. Track your steps, take the stairs, cycle to work and keep moving!

Conclusion

When losing weight, our metabolism will always slow down, making the last few pounds much harder to lose than the first few pounds.

As we age our metabolism will slow down, making weight loss at 25 far easier than weight loss at 65.

Chronic dieting will cause adaptations to your metabolism, but:

1. They are not as extreme or damaging as you may think
2. They are mostly fixable and/or avoidable with a sensible approach
3. They will not be extreme enough to prevent all progress

Calorie balance is never false but it is simultaneously simple and complicated.

While energy in versus energy out is true, a variety of factors – from energy absorption to adaptive NEAT and the thermic effect of food to slowing RMR, and even aging – can make this law feel like a continuously moving object and our body an outlier to the laws of physics.

Provided you continue to view the facts objectively and adapt accordingly, you cannot fail to achieve the goals that matter to you.

Your body can reach its best version.

FURTHER INDIVIDUALIZATION CONCLUSION

The advanced individualization methods are all short-term measures to help you make progress.

Ultimately, to *Transform for Life*, you will need to follow Lily's advice.

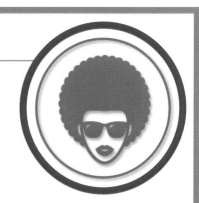

Lily's Laws

Lily just wanted to drop in and remind us of the fundamentals.

- Calorie balance
- Anabolic and catabolic flux
- Sufficient carbohydrates
- Sufficient protein
- Sufficient fat
- Drink enough water
- Eat plenty of vegetables
- Limit processed food intake
- Exercise to stimulate muscle growth and fat loss
- NEAT is an important aspect of your metabolic rate

Be compliant.
Be patient.
Be kind to yourself.
Be consistent.

And most importantly of all, remember Barry White and Billy Joel said it best:

You are perfect '*Just the way you are*'.

MAINTENANCE FUNDAMENTALS

The truth about maintenance

"How did you go bankrupt?" Bill asked.

"Two ways," Mike said. *"Gradually and then suddenly."*

With these profound words, Ernest Hemingway spoke of how the rich become poor - but the same sentences perfectly describe how rich *health* can ebb away.

Slowly at first, but then all at once.

For the majority of people, re-gaining weight or losing fitness does not happen overnight. At first, the methods that drove success are relaxed in a very small way.

"I'm so tired tonight, i'll put my feet up and watch TV instead of working out."

Where before, the approach was to 'do it anyway', reaping the rewards that finishing a workout brought. Now, with goals met, it is all too easy for the rules of engagement to change.

Yet, the door of discipline closes slowly.

It rarely makes the expectant slam that would wake you up to its potential loss. If it did, we wouldn't fail to miss it.

Beware the insidious nature of its disappearing act.

- Take note whenever you decide to miss a workout
- Switch your mind on to the moments that your emotions drive your eating decisions
- Stay alert to any signal of complacency

Isolated moments such as these will cause you no problems, provided you understand how easily they can turn into habits.

For 'health' is like taking a bath. It must be done daily...

It will never be 'easy'

Perhaps too many in the fitness industry are afraid to say this - fearful of scaring people away from their new 6 week health kicks and the dollars that follow them.

I do not share this fear, because I know that only by confronting truth can you truly live a life of health - and my aim for our members is perpetual health, not rapid change.

1. If you don't keep health as a priority, it will fade away - **slowly at first, and then all at once**. It can never be abused and ignored, it must constantly be nurtured.

2. When you hit your goals - maintaining results is easier physically than making progress - you don't need to train as hard and you can relax your diet.
3. It is harder psychologically - you now have to exercise and eat healthily without the obvious prizes that each week brings - lost weight, improved tone, improved fitness. This is a shift that must be overcome.

Once you hit your goals, you must see health as a requirement of life:

- Go to work to pay the bills
- Take a bath to stay clean
- Brush your teeth to avoid the dentist drill and bad breath
- Drink water to stay hydrated
- Exercise to be fit and healthy
- Eat well to be fit and healthy

If you want to be healthy for the rest of your life, you must always exercise and eat healthily. No matter how long you do it for, no matter how fit and healthy you are, will never be 'done'.

Sometimes, it will be hard and it will always require a level of sacrifice. The good news is, it's about the best sacrifice you will ever make.

Health for life

Reaching your aesthetic goal is not the end of your journey with health.

Losing weight and making progress should represent a small fraction of your lifelong participation in healthy behaviours and exercise.

One of the problems with weight loss is that healthy eating and exercise behaviours that accompany this goal are perceived as short-term measures in order to lose weight, rather than as distinct lifetime habits that are as important as going to work, having a shower and brushing our teeth.

Health is not something you can work at for a while, achieve and then forget about, it is something that should continue to be a priority for the rest of our lives.

If we treated our jobs the same way as most people treated health behaviours, it would go a little something like this.

1. Run out of money to pay bills, eat and live.
2. Get a job to pay the bills.
3. Keeping going to work until the bills are paid and we have enough money.
4. Success. Finances are in order! Quit our job.
5. Wait until we run out of money before looking for a new job.

It seems ridiculous when we look at it like this, but it's exactly how most people treat their health, which is far more valuable than money.

Everything within *Transform for Life* is designed to drive the way you view and approach health towards permanent and sustainable behaviours.

This is why healthy food ratios, enjoyment and exercise quantity are an important consideration from the start, long before maintenance is even considered.

If you are eating zero carbs and exercising for two hours a day when you achieve or arrive at your goal, the risk of returning to old behaviours in the classic 'all or nothing' cycle is significant.

If, on the other hand, your dieting habits are close to your maintenance habits, you will almost certainly retain them.

Setting new goals

There is good news.

If you have been losing an average of 1 lb (0.45 kg) a week and have now reached your goal weight, you will no longer have to create a calorie deficit in order to achieve your goal of maintenance.

You have two options:

A.   **Set new goals:** you can continue to improve your body composition and improve your fitness levels, but without an overall calorie deficit

B.   **Striking balance:** If you are happy with your weight, body composition and health you can work on building a new *Blueprint* based on lifetime health and balance.

Changing body composition

Just because you have hit your goal weight does not mean you cannot continue to improve the way your body looks if this is important to you. If you have hit your target weight but want to further improve your body composition you will need to use the calorie flux method to do this.

Remember the two fundamentals of body composition:

*   Fat loss only really happens in a calorie deficit
*   Muscle gain only really happens in a calorie surplus

Therefore being in a calorie balance never completely achieves one or the other.

Example body composition program:

Phase 1 fat loss focus

Current weight	180 lb (82 kg)
Current fat %	25%
Current fat weight	45 lb (20 kg)
Daily calorie requirements	2,100 kcal
Fat loss calorie intake	2,100 kcal x 0.8 = **1,680** kcal per day **
Cardio sessions per week	4 x 45 minutes
Resistance sessions per week	2 x 45 minutes
Duration	4 weeks *
Target fat loss	3 lb (1.3 kg)
Target fat percentage	23.5%
Target total fat mass	42 lb (19 kg)
Target weight	177 lb (80 kg)

Phase 2 muscle focus

Current weight	177 lb (80 kg)
Current non-fat %	76.5%
Current non-fat weight	136 lb (62 kg)
Daily calorie requirements	2,100 kcal
Muscle building calorie intake	2,100 kcal x 1.2 = **2,520** kcal per day **
Cardio sessions per week	2 x 45 minutes
Resistance sessions per week	4 x 45 minutes
Duration	6 weeks *
Target muscle gain	3 lb (1.3 kg)
Target non-fat percentage	77%
Target fat percentage	23%
Target non-fat weight	139 lb (63 kg)
Target weight	180 lb (82 kg)

* The period of time spent in muscle building is longer as muscle is usually slower to build than fat is to burn
** Calorie deficit is higher than surplus as it is usually slower for the body to build muscle than burn fat.

This is not always the case and it is important you monitor the changes in your own body.

- Body fat as a percentage continues to decrease in both phases.
- The changes are not dramatic but they are specific.
- More resistance was completed when building muscle and more cardio when stripping fat.
- The process can be lengthened to eight weeks if you have sufficient fat you can lose (more than 15% body fat in males and more than 23% body fat in females)
- The process can be repeated several times until you reach your desired fat levels
- 'Flux' can still be used within the weeks (as per flux guidelines in *The Blueprint* provided the overall calorie position is maintained

You can use *Your Health Blueprint* guidelines to build a new program based on your body composition goals.

Striking balance

If you have reached your weight loss and body composition goals and feel happy with your body you can now look at your *Blueprint* to decide on where you can make changes towards a more balanced life.

These are going to be subtle changes, with sustainability as the most important aspect of your new plan.

Let's compare a progress *Blueprint* with a maintenance blueprint.

Plan comparisons : Healthy eating

	Healthy eating	Unhealthy eating
Healthy eating ratio progress	90%	10%
Healthy eating ratio maintenance	80 %	20%

Where before better health was the priority, now sustainable health is the priority.

Health can not be sustained if we remove the predominance of healthy foods, but in maintenance the ratio can be less strict and allow for more relaxation in the overall plan.

Exercise

Days per week of exercise progress	6
Days per week of exercise maintenance	5
Exercise per day progress	45 minutes
Exercise per day maintenance	45 minutes

In this example the amount of exercise is almost the same, with just one day less overall.

Exercise is always important and retaining a high level of exercise is important to long-term goals. Maintenance always suffers when exercise is neglected.

Daily calories progress	1,750 kcal
Daily calories maintenance*	2,100 kcal

* Reverse dieting to a new calorie level is a better option than a sharp rise in your calorie levels. See chapter on *Reverse dieting* for details.

Where before the calories were set for weight loss, they are now set for maintaining weight, which means you can eat more of them. You will never be able to resume eating what you like, when you like, but rather finding a place in your life for enjoying your food, moving your body and striking the balance between health, socializing and life that works for you.

This is why it is so important you are focused on sustainable and enjoyable habits from the word go.

You can use *Your Health Blueprint* guidelines to build a new program based on your maintenance goals.

To track or not to track

By the time you reach your goal weight you should have a good idea of how many calories and macronutrients are in foods. In most instances it is perfectly feasible to stop tracking and use your instinct and improved hunger and satiety signalling to eat a balanced and healthy diet.

Some people like to track in perpetuity, but the great majority who have spent weeks and months learning how their body works and the macronutrient quantities of foods do not find it is necessary in order to maintain weight.

The 'wall weight'

Your weight will never stay exactly the same. It will fluctuate by 15 lb (7 kg) or even up to 20 lb (9 kg). The goal should be to remain with a weight range rather than at a specific weight.

Example: If your weight goal was 180 lb (82 kg), your range may be between 175-190 lb (79-86 kg).

If your weight is important to you, you can't let go of the scales entirely but should only step on them monthly or bi-weekly to keep an eye.

If you set a 'wall weight' this is the highest weight you are willing to hit before rebounding back towards your healthy range.

TASK

Decide on a wall weight.

Once you have hit the wall you can move into a short progress period to get yourself back to your maintenance weight.

You can expect to hit your wall. It does not signal failure, just an unavoidable period of imbalance that can easily be corrected.

The wall is your protection against returning to old behaviours.

Intuitive eating and movement

Maintenance is where intuitive eating comes into its own.

Learning to listen and respond to hunger, manage quantity and quality of food alongside regular movement, without the need to overthink or have to track, is the ideal scenario.

Having habits around NEAT, daily exercise, water consumption and food intake will allow you to intuitively adjust intake and output throughout your life.

Your Blueprint is phase one. It gives you the information you need to calibrate your intuition.

Once you have met your targets, with a calibrated intuition and healthy habits instilled into your life, it's time to go and live it.

Conclusion

Health is like bathing, it has to be done daily or the benefits wear off.

Expecting an extreme quick fix to get you healthy for life is like expecting to stay clean for months because you took a really long bath!

There are two philosophies that are critical to a lifetime transformation.

1. I endeavour to take pleasure in the gift of moving and nourishing my body.
2. Health is a non-negotiable part of my life. When I'm not enjoying it, I get it done anyway.

You will need both philosophies at various points in your life.

Provided you can keep them both, you will be *Transformed for Life*.

ADDITIONAL RESOURCES

TRACKERS

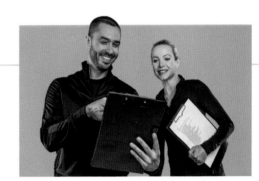

Trackers are forms to support compliance in various aspects of your health journey.

- Food compliance tracker
- Exercise compliance tracker
- Soft metrics tracker

Food compliance tracker

> **To follow the COMPLIANCE sheet is simple.**
>
> 1. Decide when you are going to eat 'healthy' based on your ratio.
> 2. Decide on when you are going to eat 'unhealthy' based on your ratio.
> 3. Put a Y in the box if you eat according to YOUR PLAN (including 'non' healthy meals).
> 4. Put an X in the box if you eat a meal or snack that was not part of your plan.
> 5. Put an O in the box if you miss a meal or snack on your plan.
> 6. Put an N/A in the box if one of the meals is not on your plan.

Day	Meal one	Snack	Meal two	Snack	Meal three
Monday					
Tuesday					
Wednesday					
Thursday					
Friday					
Saturday					
Sunday					

Exercise compliance tracker

Below are 50 squares. Every time you exercise colour one in. Write a reward on the bottom of the page and put it somewhere you can see it every day. Once it is full, 50 workouts later, go get your reward from the bottom of the page.

1		2		3		4		5	
6		7		8		9		10	
11		12		13		14		15	
16		17		18		19		20	
21		22		23		24		25	
26		27		28		29		30	
31		32		33		34		35	
36		37		38		39		40	
41		42		43		44		45	
46		47		48		49		50	

Reward

Soft metrics tracker

Tracking soft metrics will enable you to keep an eye on factors that are critical to your results but are not so concrete.

Hunger levels – How hungry do you feel through the day? 1- 5
    1 – Not hungry at all
    5 – Hungry all the time

Cravings – How often did you experience cravings? 1- 5
    1 – Not at all
    5 – Most of the time

Energy levels – How were your energy levels today? 1-5
    1 – Lots of energy
    5 – No energy at all

Mood – How was your emotional state today? 1-5
  1 – Very good
  5 – Not good at all

Sleep quality – How did you sleep? 1 -5
  1 – Very well
  5 – Not well at all

Soft Metrics Tracker:

	Mon	Tue	Wed	Thur	Fri	Sat	Sun	Total
Hunger	1	1	5	3	3	4	2	19
Cravings	2	1	5	3	4	3	2	20
Energy	3	1	3	2	2	2	2	16
Emotions	4	1	5	4	5	1	2	22
Sleep	4	2	5	4	4	5	2	26
Total	14	6	24	15	18	15	10	

What we can learn

- Tuesday and Sunday were good days.
- What were we eating Saturday and Sunday?
- Were we exercising less or more on these days?
- Wednesday was a very bad day.
- What were we eating Tuesday and Wednesday?
- Sleep is particularly bad overall. Why did we sleep well on Tuesday and Sunday?

By analysing your behaviours against these soft metrics, over time you will notice patterns that you can replicate.

Soft Metrics Tracker example:

	Mon	Tue	Wed	Thur	Fri	Sat	Sun	Total
Hunger								
Cravings								
Energy								
Emotions								
Sleep								
Total								

Behaviour tracker

Tracking behaviours gives you a proactive focus around the things you are doing and a daily victory to accompany them.

Using the behaviour tracker is easy. Tick in the box to confirm you have completed the task for that day.

	Monday	Tuesday	Wednesday	Thursday	Friday	Saturday	Sunday
Workout							
NEAT Steps							
Breakfast							
Lunch							
Dinner							
Snacks							
Avoid emotional eating							
Water							

10 Principles of Intuitive Eating

1. Reject the diet culture
Be healthy. Stop dieting.

2. Respect Your Hunger
If you feel hungry then it is fine to eat.

3. Make Peace with Food
Food is not good or bad. It is food.

4. Reject the Food Police
You are not good if you eat healthily and you are not bad if you don't.

5. Respect Your Fullness
Observe the signs that tell you you've had enough.

6. Enjoy satisfaction
Eat food guilt free, and enjoy and experience it.

7. Listen to your feelings without using foods
Food won't solve any problem except hunger.

8. Accept your genetic *Blueprint*
Your body type is your body, learn to love it.

9. Exercise
Move your body, your body loves movement.

10. Nourish your body
Eat foods that heal your body and eat foods that delight your tastebuds.

10 principles based on the intuitive eating system developed by Evelyn Tribole and Elyse Resch, founders of intuitive eating.

THE QUICKSTART GUIDE

The Blueprint is an in-depth health program designed for very specific and permanent results. If you are less concerned with specific outcomes and want a more convenient and easy to implement solution *The Quickstart Guide* is your ideal solution.

It requires less time, no tracking and can be implemented immediately.

    A.   We will help you choose an exercise plan.
    B.   Follow the exercise plan.
    C.   Make small but effective changes to your diet and lifestyle as suggested

Even though *The Quickstart Guide* is a much lighter option than *The Blueprint*, you can be confident you will:

- Lose fat and retain muscle mass
- Get fit
- Tone your muscles
- Improve most health markers
- Reduce chance of disease

If you hit a plateau and don't get results or want more specific outcomes with a tailored and definitive plan, you can create your *Blueprint* in the future.

We will help you choose an exercise plan, make small nutrition changes and improve your mental approach to health in the *Quickstart Guide*.

Quick start guide step by step guide

STEP 1: THE FITNESS TEST (OPTIONAL)

You can take the fitness test on our website by visiting the following link:

www.teambodyproject.com/fitness-test

STEP 2: CHOOSE A WORKOUT PROGRAM

    A.   If you take part in our fitness test we will recommend a workout program for you
    B.   You can choose a workout program by visiting our website

www.teambodyproject.com/workout-program

    C.   You can choose an alternative workout system by following the advice we offer on page 156 in *The Blueprint*.

STEP 3: INCREASE NEAT

Visit 159 in *The Blueprint* to learn more about why and how you should increase your daily activity levels beyond exercise.

STEP 4: TAKE MEASUREMENTS

Taking your measurements will allow you to track your progress. Visit Page 193 in *The Blueprint*.

STEP 5: GETTING EQUIPPED

You don't need much equipment, but having your set up ready will make your journey much smoother. Visit Page 195 in *The Blueprint*.

STEP 6: IMPLEMENT THE 10 RULES OF NUTRITION, EXERCISE AND MINDSET

The basics of exercise nutrition and mindset will generate 80% of the results - so the Quickstart Guide neatly outlines them.

Ten nutrition BASICS

The ten basic principles outlined below can be applied to successfully achieve results.

1. Eat protein

Most people don't eat enough protein, but protein is the building blocks of the human body. Without it we can't repair or build new muscles.

TASK

Make 25% + of each meal protein based.

2. Eat healthy fats with every meal.

Healthy fats are vital for your immune system and your emotional and physical health.

TASK

Make 25% + of each meal fats based.

3. Eat healthy carbs with every meal.

Carbs aren't bad. They support performance, energy and repair.

TASK

Make 25% + of each meal carbohydrates based.

4. Load up with vegetables.

Vegetables feel up the digestive tract, making you feel full while being packed with vitamins and minerals.

TASK

Make between a quarter and half of your plate vegetables with every meal.

5. Drink enough water.

Think you're hungry? You may be thirsty. Drink plenty of water and keep hunger at bay whilst supporting just about every process in the body.

TASK

Drink between 1 and 3 litres of water every day - adjusting for exercise, climate and overall body weight.

6. Eat slowly.

If you eat slowly you will eat less, enjoy the food more and utilise more of the nutrients.

TASK

Put your cutlery down between each mouthful and enjoy your food. Don't pick up your cutlery again until you have finished your mouthful.

7. Consider quantity.

Calorie balance drives fat and weight loss.

TASK

You can track calories, practise portion control or eat intuitively, but you must consider quantity to lose weight.

8. PLAN to break the above rules.

When it comes to weight loss, good enough is better than perfect. This creates long-term sustainability. You can't eat healthy ALL the time.

TASK

Decide when you are going to relax and break the rules. Provided you eat healthily more than 70% of the time, you will get results.

9. Control your environment.

A healthy environment makes eating healthily much easier.

TASK

Prepare your meals in advance. Have healthy snacks, water and supplements available and ready. Clear out your cupboards.

10. Food is only food

Food is all crucial for our healthy and living a good life. No food is good or bad, it is only food.

TASK

Remind yourself that food is not the solution to or cause of our problems. It is food that can be enjoyed and helps us live a healthy, happy life.

Follow these 10 rules alongside a regular exercise routine and lifelong results are guaranteed to be yours.

ACTION

Implement these rules into your health plan as much as you can.

Additional reading:

Read these chapters from *The Science* section to develop the knowledge required to get the most out of your nutrition plan.

Chapter 1 – Fundamentals of Fat Loss
Chapter 2 – Carbohydrates and
metabolic flexibility
Chapter 3 – The role of protein

Chapter 4 – Fat and ratios
Chapter 5 – Is a calorie a calorie?
Chapter 8 – Popular diets

Ten Exercise BASICS

Use the following basic rules to get the most from your exercise:

1. **Exercise for more than 150 minutes per week** to place your body in 'fat burning, muscle repairing mode' (around 20 minutes a day).

2. **Exercise for no more than 450 minutes per week** unless you have performance specific goals (around 60 minutes a day).

3. **Include a mix of resistance, cardio, mobilization and active recovery** for best results.

4. **Have at least one rest day** (total or active) per week.

5. **Have a 'lighter' exercise week every 6-8 weeks** to maximize long-term progress.

6. **Increase personal intensity** on days you have the energy.

7. **It's fine to 'go through the motions'** on days you feel tired.

8. **Know which muscles you are using** at all times.

9. **Consciously apply tension to the muscles you are working.**

10. **Just press play.** When in doubt – just do it!

ACTION

Implement these rules into your health plan as much as you can.

Additional reading:

Read the following chapters to develop the knowledge required to get the most out of your daily exercise.

Section II The Science. Chapter 6 – Understanding exercise
Section II The Science. Chapter 7 – The Importance of NEAT
Section IV The Blueprint. Chapter 2 – Choosing your workout plan

www.teambodyproject.com/additional-resources

Ten Compliance BASICS

The most important factor behind your success is getting it done. A good health plan that can be followed all of the time is infinitely better than a 'perfect' plan that you struggle to follow half the time.

1.   Just do it. THE motto at Team Body Project.

Raining? Do it anyway. Feel bad? Do it anyway. Feel tired? Do it anyway.

Nobody regretted a workout. Ever. Nobody regretted a healthy meal. Ever.

2.   Choose discipline. (Motivation is a dirty word here..)

If you think motivation will help you reach your goals - you won't reach your goals. Only discipline can help you achieve your goals.

Choose to be disciplined and see your plan through.

3.   Let 'mistakes' go.

You will make 'mistakes'. You will eat the wrong foods and miss workouts.

Provided you let it go and move on it won't have ANY impact on your results.

4.   Focus on building habits.

Habits drive everything, from drinking water and daily exercise to that Soy Latte you drink every day on the way to work.

Regular habits are the game changers.

5.   Plan 'unhealthy' meals.

You can't eat 'healthy' all the time. You decide when you do and when you don't. Be in charge of your choices, healthy and less healthy.

6.   Plan rest periods and downtimes.

You can't exercise at the limit all the time. Decide when you will put your feet up for a few days in advance.

7.   Expect peaks and troughs in your results.

There will be weeks when you don't lose weight. There will be weeks when you gain a little weight. It is inevitable. If it happens a couple of weeks in a row make some changes.

8.   Draw a line in the sand.

Every day is a new day. Bring your successes, and learn from your mistakes - don't bring them with you.

9.   **Be prepared.**

If you want to eat healthy and exercise, you have to be prepared. Prepare snacks, prepare meals and prepare your day.

10.   **Just do it. Did I say that already?**

If all else fails. Just. Do. It. This philosophy works!

You'll feel better and ready to go again if you just do it!

ACTION

Implement these rules into your health plan as much as you can.

Additional reading:

If compliance is your biggest challenge, you can learn more in the following chapters:

Section III The Art. All chapters

Join the community

Our community is made up of thousands of people who have experienced or are going through the exact same experiences as you.

This powerful community will support you, answer your questions, make you laugh and share the journey of health with you.

- The Team is a place of support, encouragement, sharing and teamwork.
- The Team is a judgement-free zone!
- The Team is a clique-free zone! Everybody is welcome and equal here from day one!
- The Team is a place of sharing knowledge, experience and lessons learned.
- The Team is a place you can be open about things you are struggling with and expect helpful guidance.

The team is most active on facebook, where the vast majority of our members interact:

www.teambodyproject.com/groups/tbpmembers

Please do introduce yourself, I can assure you will receive a warm welcome to the team.

You can also introduce yourself to the community inside our website:

www.teambodyproject.com/groups/activity

Summary

To implement a comprehensive and effective Quickstart:

- Take the fitness test (optional)
- Select a workout plan
- Focus on achieving higher NEAT
- Take measurements to track against
- Get equipped
- Implement the nutrition basics
- Implement the exercise basics
- Implement the compliance basics
- Join the community (optional)

Refer to *Transform for Life*

As you move through your experience you will have questions that arise.

You can use the information within *Transform for Life* that will support your journey.

Start the *The Blueprint* plan at any time

In the early stages of your health journey, the *Quickstart* will be enough to ensure results. If health is your overall goal it will always be enough.

If you have specific weight loss or physical goals, you may need to create a more detailed and tailored plan.

If results stop or stall, you can start the full *Transform for Life* program and find your own *Health Blueprint* for life.

HEALTHY NUTRITION

This healthy nutrition handbook will help you fill your cupboards with healthy foods and follow shopping lists that will support your health changes.

Content list

1.   Updating your cupboards
2.   Healthy shopping list
3.   Healthy vegan/plant based shopping list
4.   Snack switchers
5.   Recipe examples and daily meal planners

Updating Your Cupboards

What are processed foods?

The fewer stages of processing a food has been through, the closer it is to its original state and the more nutrients and fibre it retains.

Non-processed foods tend to be 'nutrient dense' and satiating, offering numerous benefits per calorie consumed.

On the other hand, if a food has been through more than a stage or two of processing, with each stage it tends to lose the quality of nutrient density and fibre. These types of foods are 'calorie dense'. They offer far fewer nutrients per calorie consumed, which makes them quicker to digest with less nutrient provision. This is why we tend to overeat them.

Despite what some experts claim, there is nothing wrong with eating some processed foods in your diet, provided they are not the mainstay of it.

Clearing your cupboards

We do not suggest that any food is 'bad' and everything can be eaten in moderation, however, if you are trying to make changes, being surrounded by certain foods all the time may not be a good idea.

An 'externally controlled' environment of healthy food is important as you develop the 'internal control' to live in and around all foods and enjoy them in moderation.

If you clear your cupboards of the following foods, you'll make eating healthily much easier.

Soft drinks and juices

High calorie drinks will bust your results faster than anything else. Don't drink your calories and you'll make life an awful lot easier.

Replace with: Water and teas.

Commercial Dips and Dressings: More wasted calories.

Replace with: Make your own or use spices and seasonings instead.

Processed meat: Check the label. Many processed meats contains high levels of salt, bad fats and even sugar. Eating processed meats is linked to cancer.

Replace with: Stick with the real stuff!

Microwave meals: Check the labels, but most of them contain high levels of salt, bad fats and sugar.

Replace with: Anything that is made by you!

Ice cream: Lots of sugar and easy to overeat. A great occasional treat, but if it's too tempting, get it out.

Replace with: Frozen fruit berries topped with a little natural yogurt.

Crisps, potato chips, cookies, pretzels: Salt, sugar and moorish – rarely good daily choices.

Replace with: Seeds, kale chips, homemade healthy snack bars

White foods (bread, pasta, rice): Lower fibre and less nutrient dense than whole grain counterparts.

Replace with: Brown versions.

Morning cereals: Your aim is to get a healthy macronutrient ratio in every meal, sugary cereals usually bring refined carbs and not much else.

Replace with: Oats mixed with some healthy nuts, they make a great breakfast.

Candy, cakes and chocolate: Great treats, but if you know you can't have just one piece, remove the temptation until you've got your eating discipline under control.

Replace with: 90% varieties, homemade healthy snack bars.

Healthy Shopping List

Take this list with you the next time you go shopping and you'll come away with 100% healthy ingredients.

Proteins

Meat-based Protein

- Chicken
- Turkey
- Beef
- Lean burgers and meatballs
- Steaks
- Venison

Fish-based Protein

- Wild Salmon
- Tuna
- Cod
- Roughy
- Haddock
- Shellfish
- Mackerel
- Seabass

Dairy-based Protein

- Cottage cheese
- Ricotta
- Greek cheese
- Natural and unsweetened yogurt
- Eggs

Alternative Protein Sources

- Tempeh
- Marinated tofu
- Seitan
- Chickpeas

Protein Powders

- Whey protein powders
- Vegetable protein powders
- Rice protein powders
- Pea protein powders

Note: See our 'non meat-based' proteins section to bump up the protein quantity of your meals.

Fats

Oils

- 100% pure organic butter
- Avocado spread
- Nut butters
- Coconut oil
- Olive oil
- Avocado oil
- Sesame oil
- Guacamole
- Chilli sauce

Nuts

- Walnuts
- Brazils
- Almonds
- Hazelnuts
- Pecans
- Pinenuts

Carbohydrates

Vegetables and Fresh Herbs

Buy all fresh in-season vegetables.

- Broccoli
- Carrots
- Kale
- Sweetcorn
- Cabbage
- Fennel
- Beetroot
- Peppers
- Bok choy
- Spinach

Starches

- Potatoes
- Sweet Potatoes

Grains

- Brown rice
- Buckwheat
- Bulgur
- Barley
- Millet
- Teff
- Wild Rice
- Wheat
- Amaranth
- Kamut

- Oats
- Freekeh
- Spelt

Legumes

- Lentils
- Aka beans
- Butter beans
- Cannellini beans
- Kidney beans
- Broad beans

Fruit

Any and all fresh in-season fruits.

Extras

For the Cupboard and Refrigerator

- Apple cider vinegar or other vinegars
- Soba noodles
- Sun-dried tomatoes
- Olives
- Roasted red peppers in the jar

- Cartons of kitchen ready low-salt organic ground tomatoes
- Wholewheat flour
- Artichokes in water in a jar
- Chickpea flour

Seasoning

- Red pepper flakes
- Low-sodium tamari or soy sauce
- Dried basil
- Dried oregano
- Dried rosemary
- Dried thyme
- Ground chipotle
- Chili powder
- Cumin
- Onion powder
- Ground ginger

Sweeteners

- Honey
- Agave
- Unprocessed stevia

- 100% organic maple syrup
- Blackstrap molasses

Condiments and Dips

- Non-GMO ketchup
- Mustard
- Soy or tamari sauce
- Mint sauce
- Amino acids
- Green and red pesto
- Hummous

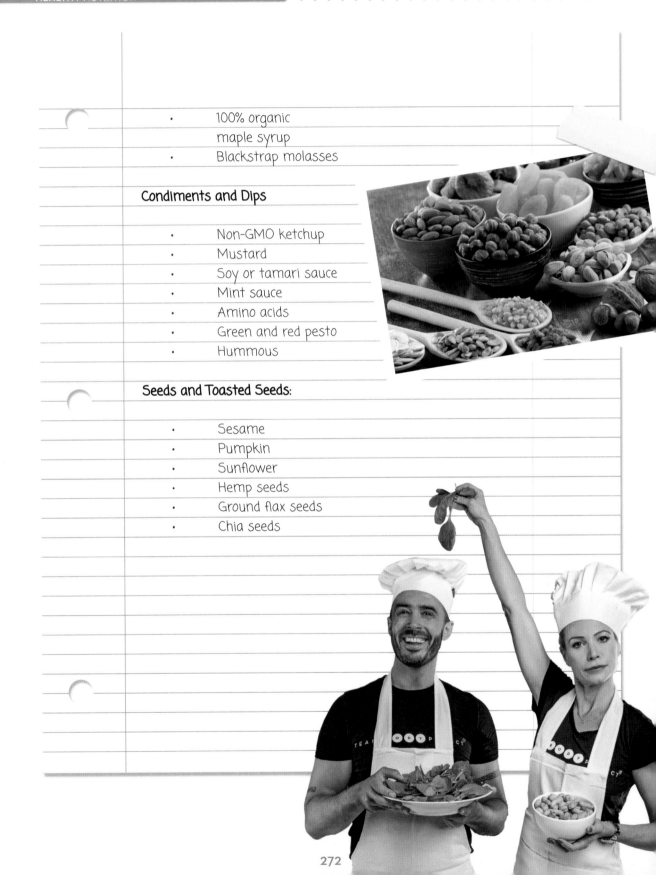

Seeds and Toasted Seeds:

- Sesame
- Pumpkin
- Sunflower
- Hemp seeds
- Ground flax seeds
- Chia seeds

Healthy Vegan/Plant Based Shopping List

Take this list with you the next time you go shopping and you'll come away with 100% healthy ingredients.

Proteins

Note: Percentage of protein in brackets.

Powders

- Soy protein powder (80%)
- Rice protein powder (77%)
- Pea protein powder (77%)
- Hemp protein powder (45%)

Legumes

- Veggie burgers (50%)
- Tofu (40%)
- Tempeh (34%)
- Lentils (30%)
- Edamame (30%)
- Peas (26%)
- Kidney beans (25%)

Grains

- Sprouted grain bread 20%
- Oats 17%
- Amaranth 16%
- Quinoa 14%

High protein vegetables

- Spinach (39%)
- Asparagus (34%)
- Broccoli (27%)
- Squash (24%)
- Seaweed (20%)

Nuts and seeds

- Hemp seeds (27%)
- Pumpkin seeds (23%)
- Flaxseeds (17%)
- Almonds and walnuts (14%)

Other high protein vegetable sources:

Beans, Seitan, Soy, Chickpeas, Green Peas, Artichokes, Chia Seeds, Hemp Milk, Black-Eyed Peas, Green Beans, Spirulina, Tahini, Nutritional Yeast, Peanut Butter, and Amaranth all have high amounts of protein.

Fats

Nuts

- Walnuts
- Brazils
- Almonds
- Hazelnuts
- Pecans
- Pinenuts

Seeds and Toasted seeds

- Sesame
- Pumpkin
- Sunflower
- Hemp seeds
- Ground flax seeds
- Chia seeds

Milk Substitutes

- Hemp milk
- Soy milk
- Almond milk
- Cashew milk
- Rice milk
- Oat milk

Yogurt

Any non-dairy yogurt including soy, almond or coconut.

Some non-dairy milks are fortified with B12. Check the label.

Carbohydrates

Vegetables and Fresh Herbs

- Broccoli
- Carrots
- Kale
- Sweetcorn
- Cabbage
- Fennel
- Beetroot
- Peppers
- Bok choy
- Spinach
- Fresh parsley
- Basil
- Coriander
- Cilantro
- Garlic
- Ginger
- Mint
- Chilli pepper

Whole Grains

- Quinoa
- Brown rice
- Barley, millet
- Teff
- Wild rice
- Wheat
- Amaranth
- Buckwheat
- Bulgar

- Kamut
- Oats

Legumes

- Lentils
- Aka beans
- Butter beans
- Cannellini beans
- Kidney beans
- Broad beans

Fruit and Frozen Fruit

Any and all fresh in-season organic fruits.

Combine them with seeds or a sprinkle of nuts.

Extras

For the Cupboard and Refrigerator

- Nutritional yeast
- Coconut oil
- Olive oil
- Avocado oil
- Sesame oil

- Apple cider vinegar
- Soba noodles
- Sun-dried tomatoes
- Olives
- Roasted red peppers in the jar
- Cartons of kitchen ready low-salt organic ground tomatoes
- Whole-wheat flour
- Artichokes in water in a jar
- Chickpea flour

Seasonings

- Red pepper flakes
- Low-sodium tamari or soy sauce
- Rice vinegar
- Dried basil
- Dried oregano
- Dried rosemary
- Dried thyme
- Ground chipotle
- Chilli powder
- Cumin
- Onion powder
- Ground ginger

Sweeteners

- Unprocessed stevia
- 100% organic maple syrup (my favourite sweetener for recipes)
- Blackstrap molasses

Condiments and Dips

Vegan mayonnaise
Non-GMO ketchup
Vegan mustard

- Vegan tamari sauce
- Mint sauce
- Amino acids
- Vegan green and red pesto
- Hummous
- Guacamole

B12 - Can be taken as a supplement, a vegetable yeast spread, in fortified cereals and grains

PROTEIN POWDER

Why so much protein?

Higher protein diets lead to more muscle gain and retention, protein costs more calories to digest and utilise, and it is the most satiating (filling) of the macronutrients - driving lower overall calorie consumption.

In short, higher protein diets result in more fat loss, more muscle retention, more sustainable results and better performance. So while we can agree getting more in our diets is a good idea, why would we choose a powder over the consumption of rich whole foods?

Are whole foods better than protein powders?

Whole foods will generally have more nutrients alongside the benefit of being unprocessed, so if you can get all of your nutrients from whole foods this would be ideal. However, 'Ideal' and the reality of life seldom meet in the middle.

Why would we choose to have a protein powder?

1. **Convenience** - It is so much quicker to prepare and drink a shake than an entire meal.
2. **Ease** - without preparation, planning and hard work, getting higher levels in the diet can be a real challenge - especially for vegetarians and vegans.

While we understand powders are not for everybody, there is no doubt that meeting a protein target with busy lives is much easier if we do up protein levels through the use of supplementation. Provided most of your diet is made up of whole foods, taking a powder to increase levels in the diet is an excellent idea.

So, if you are looking to use a powder which one should you use?

As with everything we do at Team Body Project, rather than telling you what to do, we educate you to make a decision that works for you.

Is your goal fat loss or muscle building?

This should drive your decision when choosing a powder.

If fat loss is your priority, then a powder low in calories and with as high a % or protein per 100 calories as possible is your best option. Higher protein varieties will contain around 100-120 calories per serving and provide somewhere around 20-25 grams of protein per scoop.

Other varieties may require 150 calories to provide 20-25 grams of protein. A higher percentage of protein in a powder will enable you to get the protein you need without adding additional calories from carbs or fat - for fat loss and weight loss this is crucial.

If, on the other hand you are looking to build muscle, you will want to look for a protein powder that has carbs to support your calorie surplus requirements and release the insulin needed to build muscle.

If you are struggling to get protein AND fat into your diet you will want to look at a protein powder that meets these demands.

You should look on the nutrition information to check what percentage of the calories are coming from each source and make your choice accordingly.

Do you have any specific nutrient needs?

Whey is an excellent choice for regular use. It contains all essential amino acids and is normally easily digested. However, If you are a vegetarian or vegan whey is not a good option because it contains dairy.

A vegetable based option, like pea, rice or hemp protein would be excellent alternatives, although this may sometimes limit your choice around specific nutrient qualities.

If you have IBS or lactose intolerance it may be wise to avoid lactose sugars and artificial sweeteners, and should you be gluten intolerant or celiac, powders with gluten should be avoided.

If it's important to **you** to have products that contain all natural ingredients, that should also be considered.

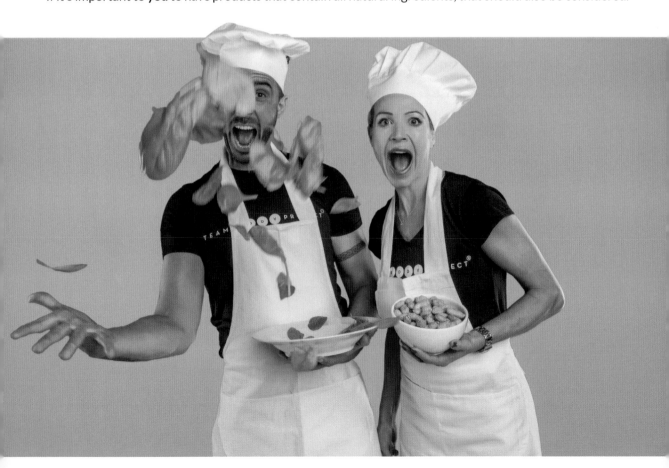

Added sugar, sweeteners and BCAA's

Unless weight gain and muscle growth is your goal added branch chain amino acids are not necessary.

Unflavoured and unsweetened varieties generally have lower sugar and sweetener levels. You can use whole foods to contribute to the taste you prefer. Peanut butter is a favourite addition of mine.

Taste and enjoyability

Lead with sustainability.

The qualities of a product are irrelevant if you don't enjoy it. There is no problem with compromising on ratios and other factors if you want a product you enjoy.

Try a few products until you find one you like.

Budget

Budget matters.

A powder that matches your needs within your budget, with 20g of protein per 120 kcals is good enough.

A powder costing twice as much with 25g of protein per 100 kcal is a little better. However it won't impact your results enough to warrant breaking your personal budget.

Provided you look to the factors that matter to you and weigh them up against each other you can make the best choice.

- Calories per g of protein
- Other macronutrient levels
- Natural ingredients or otherwise
- Sweeteners and sugars
- Specific nutrient needs
- Taste and enjoyability
- Budget

By taking these key factors into account, choosing a powder that works for you should be easy.

THE TEAM

The Team at Body Project is one of the most powerful aspects of our program. If you wish to support others as well as receive support, you will be welcomed into one of the most impressive teams on the planet!

Our community is made up of fast growing team of 6,000 people who have experienced or are going through the exact same experiences as you.

This powerful community will support you, answer your questions, make you laugh and share the journey of health with you.

The community is also a place where myself and Alexandra are able to answer member questions in real time and provide video 'question and answer' sessions and provide support.

- The Team is a place of support, encouragement, sharing and teamwork.
- The Team is a judgement-free zone!
- The Team is a clique-free zone; everybody is welcome and equal here from day one.
- The Team is a place of sharing knowledge, experience and lessons learned.
- The Team is a place you can be open about things you are struggling with and expect helpful guidance.

The team is most active on facebook, where the vast majority of our members interact:

www.teambodyproject.com/tbpmembers

Please do introduce yourself, I can assure you will receive a warm welcome to the team.

You can also introduce yourself to the community inside our website:

www.teambodyproject.com/activity

Body Project team members have been where you are and know how it feels to be at the start of a health journey.

Here are some tips some they wished somebody had told them when they started on the path to a lifetime of health.

Team tip

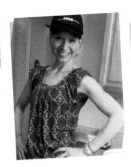

Name: Angela Vaillant Johndrow
Location: CT, USA
Age: 41
Favourite workout: Championship Boxing
Time with team: 7 months

"The rewards of TBP and our way of life are limitless. Not only do we have this unique determination and dedication, but we have the support of each other, the funny antics and laughter, and the great feeling of knowing you've done something great for your body. And if you chose not to press play, it is OK and you can try again tomorrow."

Team tip

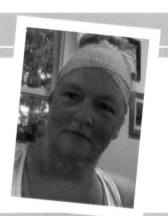

Name: Laura Van Den Eynden
Location: Ontario, USA
Age: 48
Favourite workout: Championship boxing
Time with team: 16 months

"Daniel Bartlett never commented on how bad certain foods were JUST enjoy them for what they are and move on."

Team tip

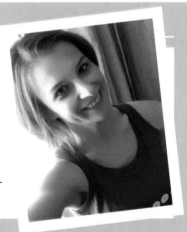

Name: Marinela Albu
Location: Romania
Age: 32
Favourite workout: Ultimate Legs
Time with team: 24 months

"Do the type of workout you enjoy and have time for. This way your body and your mind will get hooked and exercising will become non-negotiable for you."

Team tip

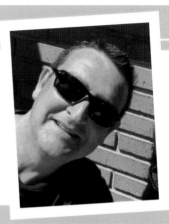

Name: Craig Fisher
Location: Villamartin, Spain
Age: 48
Favourite workout: Championship Boxing 2
Time with team: 17 months

"Press play, once a day. That's how I do it when I work away for 8 weeks at time."

Team tip

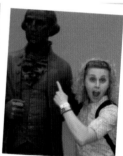

Name: Tara Chase
Location: Utah, USA
Age: 34
Favourite workout: Ultimate Tabata
Time with team: 16 months

"Something I learned on was that eating right 85-90% of the time was the key. If I do that, then the other 10-15% will not make a difference. That's really helped my approach to food and making good food choices."

Team tip

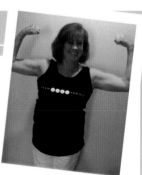

Name: Karen Rogers
Location: Stockton, California
Age: 58
Favourite workout: Cardio Starter
Time with team: 9 months

"You've got to let go of any guilt associated with putting your health first. As Daniel says, workout time is your time. What has helped me was to fully involve my family and friends. Telling them I was doing this and explaining how important it is to me.

Our community is awesome but we also need those closest in our lives to be there for us as well. To let them know I may not be able to pick up that phone or text immediately if I'm in a workout but I will get to you and with a much better ability to give you all the attention you deserve to have from me."

Team tip

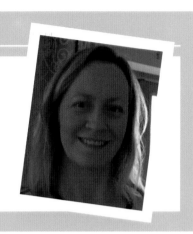

Name: Tricia McLoughlin
Location: Leitrim, Ireland
Age: 46
Favourite workout: Sparta
Time with team: 2 years

"It's your journey; you're comparing yourself only to the you of yesterday, last week, last month, last year and not to anyone else."

Team tip

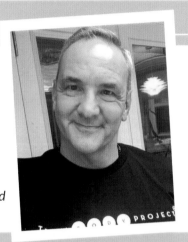

Name: Mike Fleming
Location: Georgia, USA
Age: 52
Favourite workout: Ultimate Hybrid
Time with team: 19 months

"Tell me why you didn't work out, and I'll give you the same answer as to why you should have! After it's done, I have never regretted pressing play. I have regretted, however, times I skipped it for sore excuses."

Team tip

Name: Nikki Baxter
Location: Arkansas, USA
Age: 34
Favourite workout: Interval cardio
Time with team: 4 months

"Something I have noticed is the importance of taking time for myself. In my case, it is taking the time after work to do my workouts. I can come up with a million reasons that I should be doing something else – dishes, laundry, dinner, hanging out with my sons (even though they're teenagers and probably couldn't care less about hanging out with their mom)… and what I have noticed is that during that one hour of me taking care of myself and making myself healthier, the Earth keeps spinning!

Team tip

Name: Alaine Smith
Location: France
Age: 32
Favourite workout: AvD Still Personal
Time with team: 10 months

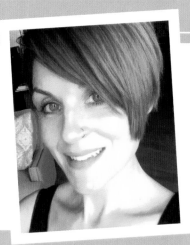

"Stop thinking of it as being 'on' or 'off' the wagon – there is no wagon!!! It's OK to have a bad day, or a bad workout. That doesn't mean the next meal or next workout has to be that way. Each day/meal is a new chance."

Team tip

Name: Fran Devlin
Location: Pinehurst, USA
Age: 38
Favourite workout: Championship Boxing 2
Time with team: 12 months

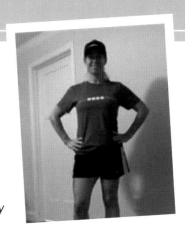

"Setting time aside and sitting down to plan what your day will look like BEFORE you eat, before you track, is so helpful, especially when you're learning what's what. It helps to plug things in and play around with the percentages without actually consuming anything, for macros and calories.

If I plug things in after I eat randomly then I tell myself I have to be objective because of all the emotional ties to it. It's too easy to get mad at myself otherwise."

Team tip

Name: John Prockter
Location: Shropshire, UK
Age: 38
Favourite workout: HIIT with Daniel
Time with team: 4 months

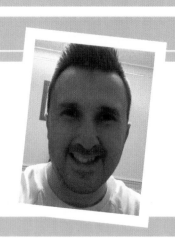

"Tell everyone you're about to work out when you really don't want to so you have to post a 'swelfie' after."

Team tip

Name: Shannon McGrath Collins
Location: Indiana, USA
Age: 34
Favourite workout: Championship Boxing 2
Time with team: 9 months

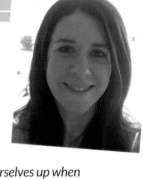

"I had several years of trying to get healthy and active that never panned out. The emotions and physical body are linked. The biggest part of this is the internal dialogue we give to ourselves. If we beat ourselves up when we miss a workout, or eat a cheat meal, or not put in as much effort as we would've liked or not hit that goal weight, it will be nearly impossible to stay on the journey to health and wellness.

You can't mentally beat yourself up and expect your physical body to reach its full potential. I've learned to treat myself as I would a friend. Be forgiving, be gentle, listen to both my body and my emotions. If you change the negative thoughts to positive things you would say to motivate a friend, it makes it so much easier to power through the rough times. Putting in the emotional work is sometimes harder than any workout I've done, but I really think it has made the difference to embracing a healthy lifestyle!"

Team tip

Name: Ben Aveling
Location: Northamptonshire, UK
Age: 32
Favourite workout: Get moving 3
Time with team: 8 months

"I don't know about you but I'm a "Flick a switch" kind of person, so find I can adjust to a new regime easily, it's normally just "for how long". But this time I believe. My advice is try to be in the journey with someone you care about and people that matter. I think that the community that engage regularly on Facebook and over on TBP.com are by far the most invaluable resource. You can be as strict as you like, lose loads of weight and have achieved amazing things but nothing feels better than having someone to tell and share. Oh, and spoons of peanut butter of course."

TRANSFORM FOR LIFE GLOSSARY OF TERMS

Adaptation: A change to your body created through overload

Anabolic: A metabolic state of building

Beep: A noise that indicates a completed rep and keeps correct speed

BMR: baseline metabolic rate

Calorie flux: A period of higher or lower calories

Calorie surplus: More calories than baseline requirements

Calorie deficit: Less calories than baseline requirement

Catabolic: A metabolic state of breakdown

Cheating reps: The use of momentum at the end of a set to overcome lactic threshold

Chronic exposure: Continuous exposure to surplus or deficit

Core: The muscles supporting the spine that support every movement

Dropping: Allowing gravity to complete a movement instead of engaging muscles

Eccentric control: Controlling a movement against gravity

Ectomorph: Body type; smaller bone structure and longer limbs

Endomorph: Body type; larger bone structure and shorter limbs

Flux: A period of higher calories to support anabolic repair and adaptation

Gluconeogenesis: Conversion of protein to glucose

Hypercaloric state: Calorie surplus

Hypocaloric state: Calorie deficit

Ketogenic diet: A diet of more than 70% fat

Lipolysis: A fat burning state

Macronutrient: Fat, carbohydrate or protein substrate

Mesomorph: Body type; medium bone structure and an athletic overall shape

Metabolic flexibility: The capacity for the individual to adapt fuel oxidation to fuel availability.

Micronutrient: Vitamins, minerals and other trace elements in food.

Momentum: A swinging movement that does not require sufficient muscular engagement

Muscular engagement: The conscious use of a muscle

NEAT: Non exercise activity thermogenesis

Reps/repetition: The amount of times you complete a 'repetition' of an exercise

Substrate: A macronutrient, fat, carbohydrate or protein

Sculptor: A 'plug-on' resistance based TBP workout

Satiety: The satisfied feeling of being full after eating

Sets: The amount of sets you can complete of a group of repetitions

Squeeze: Contraction at the 'top' of a concentric movement

Thermodynamics: a branch of physics concerned with heat and temperature and their relation to energy and work.

Thermogenesis: The process of heat production in living organisms.

Time under tension: The amount of time the muscle both with and against gravity

Tracking: The process of monitoring foods and drinks consumed against movement

Turbo: An extra workout that is designed to add to your program to accelerate results

Progression: A workout plan that constantly changes variables (applied to Sculptors)

Variable: A factor that changes and impacts results

Endnotes – Fundamentals of Fat Loss

[1] Payne P. R. and Dugdale A. E. "A Model for the Prediction of Energy Balance and Body Weight." Annals of Human Biology, 4 (1977):525–535.

[2] Payne P. R. and Dugdale A. E. "Mechanisms for the Control of Body-Weight." Lancet, 309 (1977):583–586.

[3] Hall K. D. "What is the Required Energy Deficit per Unit Weight Loss?" International Journal of Obesity, 32 (2008):573–576.

[4] Dugdale A. E. and Payne P. R. "Pattern of Lean and Fat Deposition in Adults." Nature, 266 (1977):349–351.

[5] Janssen I., et al. "Effects of an Energy-Restrictive Diet with or without Exercise on Abdominal Fat, Intermuscular Fat, and Metabolic Risk Factors in Obese Women." Diabetes Care, 25 (2002):431–438.

[6] Marniemi J., et al. "Metabolic Changes Induced by Combined Prolonged Exercise and Low-Calorie Intake in Man." European Journal of Applied Physiology and Occupational Physiology, 53 (1984):121–127.

[7] Mäestu J., et al. "Anabolic and Catabolic Hormones and Energy Balance of the Male Bodybuilders During the Preparation for the Competition." Journal of Strength and Conditioning Research, 24 (2010):1074–1081.

[8] Tipton K.D. and Ferrando, A.A. "Improving muscle mass: response of muscle metabolism to exercise, nutrition and anabolic agents." Essays in Biochemistry, (2008) 85-98.

[9] DeBerardinis and R.J., Thompson, C. B. "Cellular Metabolism and Disease: What Do Metabolic Outliers Teach Us?" Cell, 148 (2012) 1132:1144

[10] Kreitzman S. N. "Factors Influencing Body Composition During Very Low-Calorie Diets." American Journal of Clinical Nutrition, 56 (1992):217S–223S.

[11] Bopp, M. J., et al. "Lean Mass Loss Is Associated with Low Protein Intake during Dietary-Induced Weight Loss in Postmenopausal Women." Journal of the American Dietetic Association, 108 (2008) 1216:1220.

[12] Hagopian K., et al. "Long-Term Calorie Restriction Reduces Proton Leak and Hydrogen Peroxide Production in Liver Mitochondria." American Journal of Physiology Endocrinology and Metabolism, 288 (2005):E674-E684.

[13] Asami D. K., et al. "Effect of Aging, Caloric Restriction, and Uncoupling Protein 3 (UCP3) on Mitochondrial Proton Leak in Mice." Experimental Gerontology, 43 (2008):1069–1076.

[14] Tomiyama, A.J., et al. "Low Calorie Dieting Increases Cortisol." Psychosomatic Medicine, 72 (2010) 357-364.

[15] Rosenbaum M., et al. "Long-Term Persistence of Adaptive Thermogenesis in Subjects Who Have Maintained a Reduced Body Weight." American Journal of Clinical Nutrition, 88 (2008):906–912.

[16] Howard C.E. and Porzelius L.K. "The Role of Dieting in Binge Eating Disorder: Etiology and Treatment Implications." Clinical Psychology Reviews, 19 (1999): 25-44.

[17] MacLean P. S., et al. "Peripheral Metabolic Responses to Prolonged Weight Reduction That Promote Rapid, Efficient Regain in Obesity-Prone Rats." American Journal of Physiology – Regulatory, Integrative and Comparative Physiology, 290 (2006): R1577-R1588.

[18] Maclean P. S., et al. "Biology's Response to Dieting: The Impetus for Weight Regain." American Journal of Regulatory, Integrative and Comparative Physiology, 301 (2011): R581–R600.

[19] Helms and E. R., Aragon, A. A., Fitschen, P.J. "Evidence-based Recommendations for Natural Bodybuilding Contest Preparation: Nutrition and Supplementation." Journal of the International Society of Sports Nutrition, 11 (2014).

[20] Longland, T.M., et al. "Higher Compared with Lower Dietary Protein During an Energy Deficit Combined with Intense Exercise Promotes Greater Lean Mass Gain and Fat Mass Loss: a Randomized Trial." American Journal of Clinical Nutrition, 103 (2016): 738 -746.

[21] Davoodi S. H., et al. "Calorie Shifting Diet Versus Calorie Restriction Diet: A Comparative Clinical Trial Study." International Journal of Preventive Medicine 5, (2014): 447-456.

[22] Ravussin E., et al. "Energy Expenditure Before and During Energy Restriction in Obese Patients." American Journal of Clinical Nutrition, 41 (1985): 753–759.

[23] Doucet E., et al. "Evidence for the Existence of Adaptive Thermogenesis During Weight Loss." British Journal of Nutrition, 85 (2001): 715–723.

[24] Connolly, J., Romano and T., Patruno, M. "Effects of Dieting and Exercise on Resting Metabolic Rate and Implications for Weight Management." Family Practice, 16 (1999): 196–201.

[25] Weigle, D.S. "Contribution of Decreased Body Mass to Diminished Thermic Effect of Exercise in Reduced-Obese Men." International Journal of Obesity, 12 (1988): 567–578.

[26] Rosenbaum M., et al. "Long-Term Persistence of Adaptive Thermogenesis in Subjects Who Have Maintained a Reduced Body Weight." American Journal of Clinical Nutrition, 88 (2008): 906–912.

[27] Kresta, J. Y., et al. "Effects of Diet Cycling on Weight Loss, Fat Loss and Resting Energy Expenditure in Women" Journal of the International Society of Sports Nutrition, 7, Supp 1 (2007): 21.

[28] Correia-Oliveira, C. R. et al. "Strategies of Dietary Carbohydrate Manipulation and Their Effects on Performance in Cycling Time Trials." Sports Medicine, 43 (2013): 707-719.

Endnotes – Carbohydrates and Metabolic Flexibility

[1] Rorsman P. and Braun M. "Regulation of Insulin Secretion in Human Pancreatic Islets." Annual Review of Physiology, 75 (2013): 155–179.

[2] Henquin J.C. et al. "Hierarchy of the Beta-Cell Signals Controlling Insulin Secretion." European Journal of Clinical Investigation, European Journal of Clinical Investigation, 33 (2003): 742-750.

[3] Ramnanan C. J., et al. "Physiologic Action of Glucagon on Liver Glucose Metabolism." Diabetes, Obesity and Metabolism, 13 (2011): S118-125.

[4] Cooperberg, B. A. and Cryer, P.E. "Insulin Reciprocally Regulates Glucagon Secretion in Humans." Diabetes, 59 (2010): 2936–2940.

[5] Kelley D. E. "Skeletal Muscle Fat Oxidation: Timing and Flexibility Are Everything." Journal of Clinical Investigation, 115 (2005): 1699-1702.

[6] Kelley D. E., et al. "The Effect of Non-Insulin-Dependent Diabetes Mellitus and Obesity on Glucose Transport and Phosphorylation in Skeletal Muscle." Journal of Clinical Investigation 97 (1996): 2705-2713.

Endnotes – The Role of Protein

[1] Meredith C. N., et al. "Dietary Protein Requirements and Body Protein Metabolism in Endurance-Trained Men." Journal of Applied Physiology, 66 (1989) 2850-2856.

[2] Fontana L., et al. "Effect of Long-Term Calorie Restriction with Adequate Protein and Micronutrients on Thyroid Hormones." Journal of Clinical Endocrinology and Metabolism, 91 (2006): 3232-3235.

[3] Phillips S.M., Moore, D.R. and Tang, J.E. "A critical examination of dietary protein requirements, benefits, and excesses in athletes." International Journal of Sports Nutrition and Exercise Metabolism, 17 (2007): S58-76.

[4] Shultz, Y. "Protein Turnover, Ureagenesis and Gluconeogenesis." International Journal for Vitamin and Nutrition Research, 81 (2011): 101-7.

[5] Dulloo A. G. and Samec S. "Uncoupling Proteins: Their Roles in Adaptive Thermogenesis and Substrate Metabolism Reconsidered." British Journal of Nutrition 86 (2001): 123–139.

[6] Khan M.A., Gannon M.C. and Nuttall F.Q. "Glucose Appearance Rate Following Protein Ingestion in Normal Subjects." Journal of the American College of Nutrition 11 (1992): 701–706.

[7] Hoffman, J.R., Falvo and M.J. "Protein – Which is Best?" Journal of Sports Science & Medicine, 3 (2004): 118–130.

Endnotes – Fats and Ratios

[1] Wang, Y., et al. "Transcriptional regulation of hepatic lipogenesis", Nature Reviews Molecular Cell Biology, 16 (2015): 678-689.

[2] Gómez-Pinilla, F. "Brain Foods: the Effects of Nutrients on Brain Function." Nature Reviews in Neuroscience, 9 (2008): 568-578.

[3] Veldhorst M.A., Westerterp-Plantenga M.S. and Westerterp K.R. "Gluconeogenesis and Energy Expenditure After a High-Protein, Carbohydrate-Free Diet." American Journal of Clinical Nutrition, 90 (2009): 519-526.

[4] McCarthy J.J., Esser and K.A. "Anabolic and Catabolic Pathways Regulating Skeletal Muscle Mass." Current Opinion in Clinical Nutrition and Metabolic Care, 13 (2010): 230–235.

[5] Vergnaud, A.C., et al. "Macronutrient Composition of the Diet and Prospective Weight Change in Participants of the EPIC-PANACEA Study." PLoS One 8 (2013): e57300.

[6] Simopoulos, A. P. "The importance of the ratio of omega-6/omega-3 essential fatty acids." Biomedicine and Pharmacotherapy, 56 (2002): 365-379.

[7] Iqbal, M.P. "Trans Fatty Acids – A Risk Factor for Cardiovascular Disease." Pakistan Journal of Medical Sciences, 30 (2014): 194-197.

[8] Dashti, H.M., et al. "Long-Term Effects of a Ketogenic Diet in Obese Patients." Experimental & Clinical Cardiology, 9 (2004): 200-205.

Endnotes – Is a calorie a calorie

[1] Klok M.D., Jakobsdottir S. and Drent M.L. "The Role of Leptin and Ghrelin in the Regulation of Food Intake and Body Weight in Humans: A Review." Obesity Reviews, 8 (2007): 21-34.

[2] Duncan, K.H., Bacon, J.A and Weinsier, R.L. "The Effects of High and Low Energy Density Diets on Satiety, Energy Intake, and Eating Time of Obese and Nonobese Subjects." American Journal of Clinical Nutrition, 37 (1983): 763-767.

[3] Stelmach-Mardas, M. et al. "Link Between Food Energy Density and Body Weight Changes in Obese Adults." Nutrients. 8 (2016): 229.

[4] Traoret, CJ, et al. "Digestion and energy balance". International Journal of Obesity. (2008)

[5] Guangchang Pang et al "Energy intake, metabolic homeostasis, and human health" Food Science and Human Wellness 2014

[6] Hall, K.D. "Predicting metabolic adaptation, body weight change, and energy intake in humans". Am J Physiol Endocrinol Metab (2010)

[7] Jenkins D.J., et al. "Glycemic index of foods: a physiological basis for carbohydrate exchange." American Journal of Clinical Nutrition, 34 (1981): 362–6.

Endnotes – Understanding exercise

[1] Morton J.P., et al. "The exercise-induced stress response of skeletal muscle, with specific emphasis on humans." Sports Medicine, 39 (2009): 643-662.

[2] Donnely, J.E. "Position Stand: Appropriate Physical Activity Intervention Strategies for Weight Loss and Prevention of Weight Regain for Adults." Medicine & Science in Sports & Exercise, 41 (2009): 451-471.

[3] Willis, L.H., et al. "Effects of Aerobic and/or Resistance Training on Body Mass and Fat Mass in Overweight or Obese Adults." Journal of Applied Physiology, 113 (1985): 1831-1837.

[4] Grundy, S.M., et al. "Roundtable Consensus Statement: Physical Activity in the Prevention and Treatment of Obesity and its Comorbidities." Medicine & Science in Sports & Exercise, 31 (1999): 1493-1500.

[5] Ross, R., Janssen, I. "Is Abdominal Fat Preferentially Reduced in Response to Exercise-Induced Weight Loss?" Medicine & Science in Sports & Exercise 31 (1999): S568-S572.

[6] Hagan, R.D., et al. "The Effects of Aerobic Conditioning and/or Caloric Restriction in Overweight Men and Women." Medicine & Science in Sports & Exercise. 18 (1986):87-94.

[7] Myers J., et al. "Exercise Capacity and Mortality Among Men Referred for Exercise Testing." New England Journal of Medicine, 14 (2002): 793-801.

[8] Craft, L. L., Pernas, F. M. "The Benefits of Exercise for the Clinically Depressed." Clinical Psychiatry 6(2004): 104-111.

[9] Sharma, A., Madaan, V., Petty, F.D., "Exercise for Mental Health." Primary Care Companion Journal of Clinical Psychiatry. 8 (2006):106.

[10] Westcott, W.L. "Resistance Training is Medicine: Effects of Strength Training on Health." Current Sports Medicine Reports. 11 (2012): 209-16.

[11] Burd, N.A., et al. "Muscle Time Under Tension During Resistance Exercise Stimulates Differential Muscle Protein Sub-Fractional Synthetic Responses in Men." Journal of Physiology, 590 (2012): 351-362.

Endnotes – The importance of NEAT

[1] Levine, J.A., "Non-Exercise Activity Thermogenesis (NEAT)." Best Practice & Research: Clinical Endocrinology & Metabolism, 16 (2002): 679-702.

[2] Christian von Loeffelholz "The Role of Non-exercise Activity Thermogenesis in Human Obesity". Department of Clinical Nutrition, June 5, 2014.

Endnotes – Popular diets

[1] McCartney, M. "Margaret McCartney: Clean eating and the cult of healthism" British Medical Journal, 354 (2016): i4095.

[2] Westwater, M.L., Fletcher, P.C., Ziauddeen, H. "Sugar Addiction: the State of the Science." European Journal of Nutrition, 55 Supp 2 (2016): 55-69.

[3] Neurosci Biobehav Rev. 2008; "Evidence for Sugar Addiction: Behavioral and Neurochemical Effects of Intermittent, Excessive Sugar Intake." Nicole M. Avena, Pedro Rada, and Bartley G. Hoebel*

[4] Jacobsen, M.F. "Six Arguments for a Greener Diet: How a More Plant-Based Diet Could Save Your Health and the Environment". (Washington, DC: Center for Science in the Public Interest, 2006).

[5] Arun Swaminathan and Gregory A. Jicha"Nutrition and prevention of Alzheimer's dementia".
Front Aging Neurosci. 2014.

[6] Hashim, S.A., VanItallie, T.B. "Ketone Body Therapy: from the Ketogenic Diet to the Oral Administration of Ketone Ester." Journal of Lipid Research, 55 (2014): 1818-1826.

[7] Dashti, H.M., et al. "Long-Term Effects of a Ketogenic Diet in Obese Patients." Experimental & Clinical Cardiology, 9 (2004): 200-205.

[8] Roger Collier; 185(9): "Intermittent fasting: the science of going without". Jun 11 (2013): 109-4451.

Index

AFTERWORD: PROCRASTINATION

Knowledge can change your life, but only if you act on it immediately.

The longer you wait to act, the less likely change is to happen.

- The best time to start is now
- The second best time to start is a planned date in the very near the future
- The worst time to start is after/when/if

If your health matters to you, act on it at the first available opportunity.

I have witnessed remarkable individuals starting health plans through cancer treatment, when nursing relatives with terminal illnesses, during job promotions and redundancies, in the midsts of marital breakups, depression and anxiety, and through every other conceivable life challenge.

Every single one of these incredible people has said the same thing.

The time they spent on their health was returned ten times over. It was worth every moment given and compromise made.

There is no wonderful or even tragic life event that can remove the importance of taking time on our health.

Our health can and will support us physically when we are emotionally empty.

- There is no more perfect moment to start a health plan than right now
- What better moment to workout than the one you scheduled?
- Does a more suitable moment to improve your diet exist than the next meal you eat?

What are you waiting for?

Just. Do. It.

ABOUT THE AUTHORS

Team Body Project founders Daniel and Alexandra Bartlett are married and live in West London with their 3 children.

They blend Alexandra's expertise in Pilates, mobilisation and nutrition with Daniel's expertise in fitness, weight management and personal development to create a complete health product.

Team Body Project has reached over 20 million people worldwide and their website www.teambodyproject.com currently has over 11,000 active members.

They have spoken on multiple aspects of health at FTSE 500 companies and host popular health events globally.

As passionate opponents of unsubstantiated diets promising easy outcomes, they advocate a lifestyle based method that includes evidence based exercise and nutrition plans.

Everything they do is infused with their message of personal empowerment, development and self confidence.

They both enjoy a glass of wine, good food and excellent company.

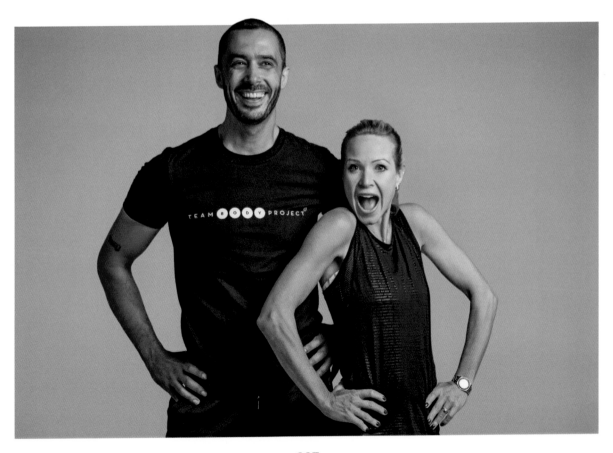

HEALTH, EXERCISE AND DIET DISCLAIMER

The health, fitness and nutritional information in this book is for educational purposes only. The use of any information provided in this book is entirely at your own risk.

You should not rely on the information in Transform for Life as a substitute for professional medical advice, diagnosis, or treatment. If you have any concerns or questions about your health, you should always consult with a physician or other health-care professional. Do not disregard, avoid or delay obtaining medical or health related advice from your health-care professional because of something you may have read in this book.

You should consult your doctor/physician or other health care professional before starting this or any other health and fitness program to determine if it is right for your needs. This is particularly true if you have a history of high blood pressure or heart disease, or if you have ever experienced chest pain when exercising or have experienced chest pain in the past month when not engaged in physical activity, smoke, have high cholesterol, are obese, or have a bone or joint problem that could be made worse by a change in physical activity. Do not make any changes to your diet or exercise plan if your physician or health care provider advises against it.

If you experience faintness, dizziness, pain or shortness of breath at any time while exercising you should stop immediately.

Developments in medical research may impact the health, fitness and nutritional advice that appears in this book.

No assurance can be given that the advice contained in this site will always include the most recent findings or developments with respect to the particular material.

NOTES

NOTES

NOTES